150 WAYS TO MAKE YOUR Dental Practice ROCK!

Arun K. Garg, DMD

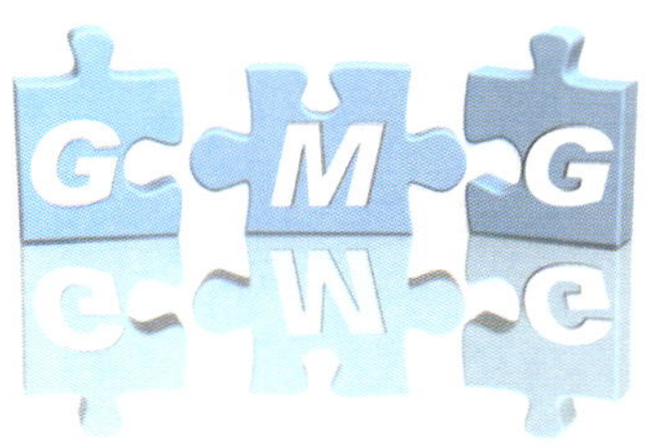

GARG MULTIMEDIA GROUP
MIAMI

Garg Multimedia Group, Inc.
1840 NE 153rd Street
North Miami Beach, FL 33162

ISBN: 978-0-9820953-6-2

Edited by Daniel Teigman
Cover and interior design by Robert Mott, RobertMottDesigns.com
Photo direction and Shutterstock.com photo licensing by Garg Multimedia Group
Printed in the United States of America by Bang Printing, Brainerd, Minnesota

First Edition

Dear Reader,

Of the many small and medium sized businesses that exist, none are as unique as a dentist's office. At the crossroads of science, art, customer service and medicine, dentistry is about tinkering with one of the most critical aspects of physical expression — the human smile. Intricate in its detail, exquisite in the information it imparts, our smiles say so much about us that it requires a significant leap of faith to let someone else — even a professional — work on our teeth.

One of the ways patients first evaluate whether they've selected the right dental practice is by a gut sense of how the office operates. From the first read of a marketing brochure, to the first phone call, to the first in-office appointment, little by little patients build a mental picture that tells them they've made the right choice, or cautions them to steer a different course.

While this method of testing the waters has its benefits, it's not foolproof. Very often a dental office's patient management has little or no correlation to the expertise of the actual dentist. How disheartening to think that a great dentist might lose a patient's business all because that patient felt they were mistreated on the phone or spoken to in a rude manner. In addition to snags like this, business management related to billing and patient files can also, over time, leave a poor (and lasting) impression.

This book, which contains 150 ways to improve your dental practice, is written with the goal of eliminating the disconnect between a dental practice's business management style and the quality of the services provided. Each tip is written in an easy-to-read conversational style. Think of them as part short story and part lively anecdote. Read them one at a time or in bulk. Make copies and encourage your staff to read the material too. I guarantee that following just a few of these tips will radically enhance your dental practice. Efficiencies will improve, patient satisfaction will increase, inter-office stress and anxiety will be reduced, and your patient base will grow.

Today dentistry is considered one of America's fastest growing and most satisfying professions. Not just for the dentist, but for his support staff as well. While such reports are encouraging, what it leaves it out is how varied the dental practice landscape truly is. Some practices are thriving and living up to these impressions while others struggle, overwhelmed by overhead and an over reliance on a patient management style that doesn't work.

Don't be one of the practices sitting on the sidelines of success. This book, and the knowledge contained within its pages, is the tool that can help reinvent your dental office. As the economy continues its post recession rebound and more patients seek dental treatment, now is the time you can help make your dental practice rock!

Happy reading!

Arun K. Garg, DMD

Overnight Success is as Unrealistic as Overnight Failure

Dental practices, like all business, take time to build their customer base. Success doesn't happen over night.

Likewise, when a dental practice struggles, especially several years into its existence, the structural flaws that gave rise to that struggle, crept up slowly. After all, if they had been noticed sooner, ideally those flaws wouldn't have been permitted to manifest.

Like a rotted tooth, once a business foundation is "infected" with poor management and marketing, it's hard to recover.

Encouragingly the reverse is also true.

Successful dental practices are the ones that remain nimble – flexible to ever-shifting local, regional and national trends.

Even if your dental practice hasn't adopted a quick-thinking mindset, it's never too late to start. Just remember, overnight success is as unrealistic as overnight failure – no matter what the media says!

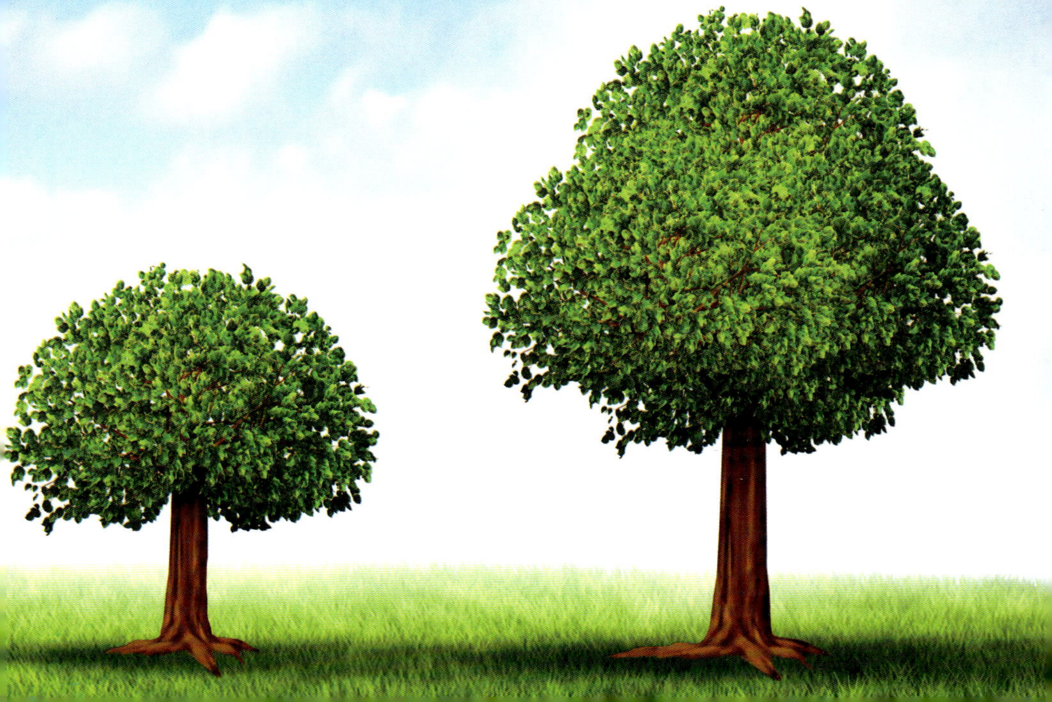

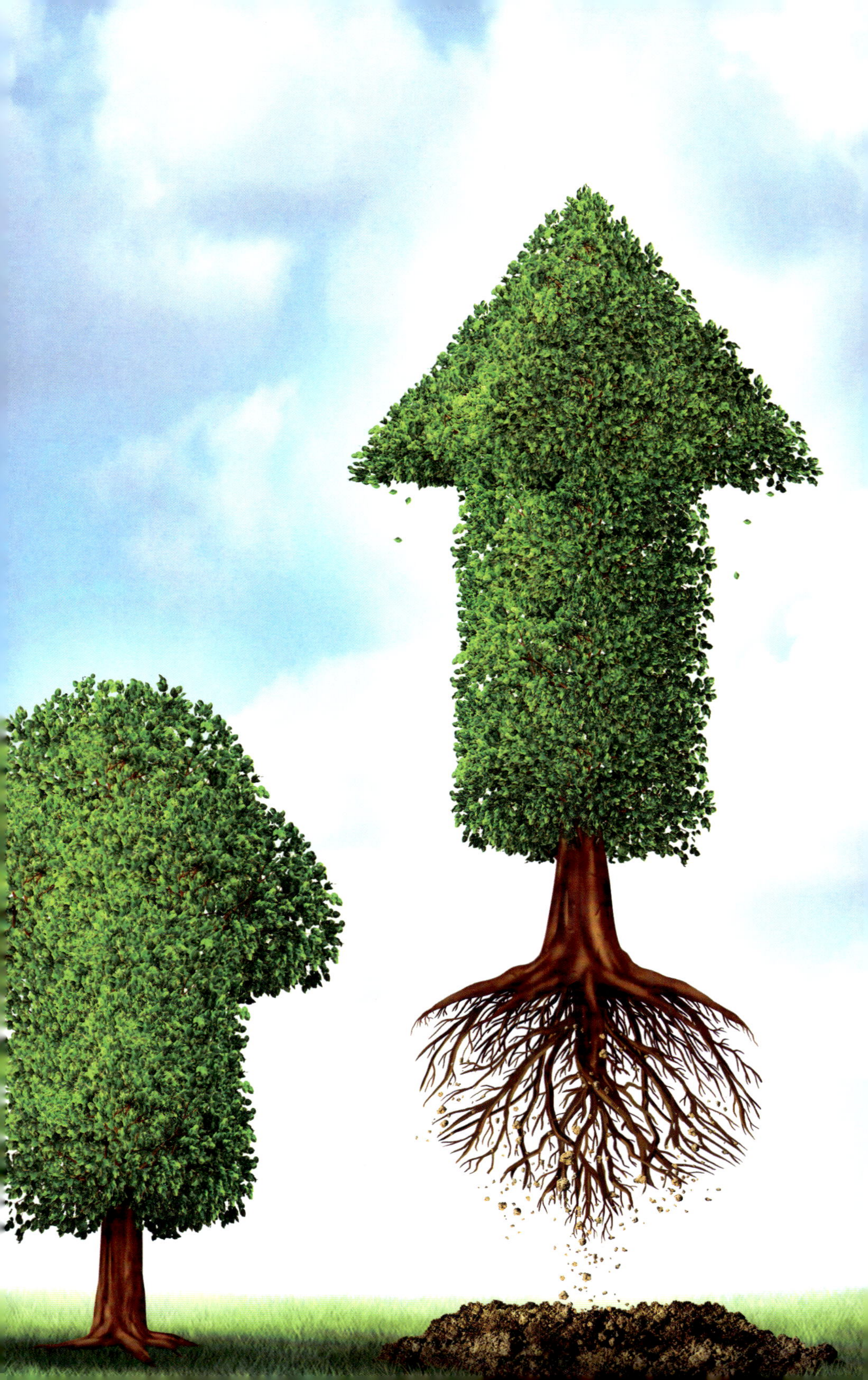

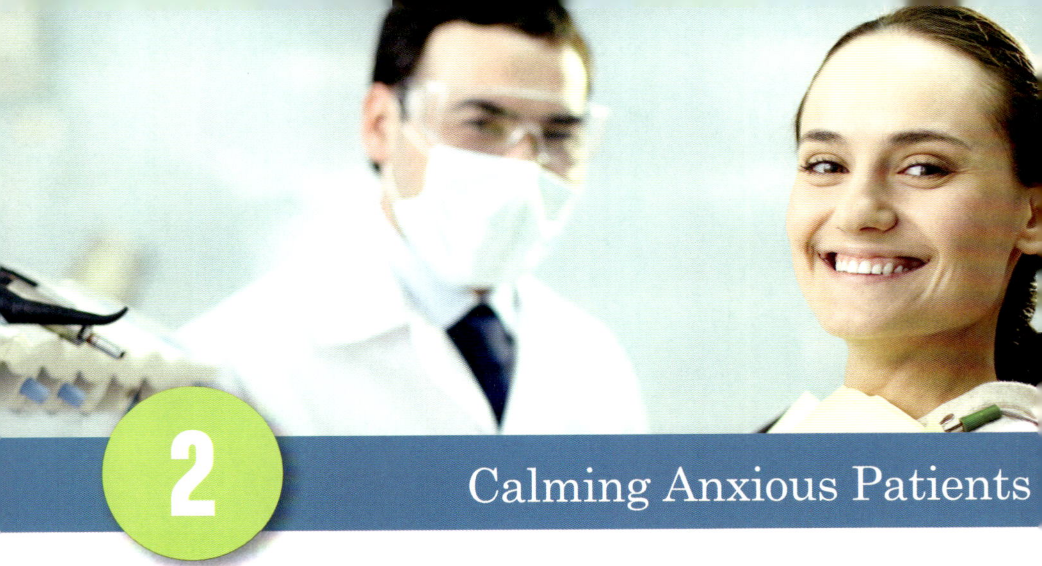

2 Calming Anxious Patients

Anxious patients are a golden opportunity to create raving fans for your practice. But they must be handled correctly. Here is one effective way:

Patient: "I'm scared to death of the dentist."

Team Member: "I appreciate you sharing your concern. That's a very normal feeling. Tell me more."

Patient: "I hate needles."

Team Member: "Thanks for telling me. Your comfort is our first concern. I will let the doctor know about your concern so she will take extra good care of you. Most of our patients mention how caring Dr. Jones is. And I will be with you the entire time."

Additional distinctions:

- Acknowledge the patients' feelings and that the feelings are valid.
- Reinforce that their comfort is your #1 priority.
- Encourage patients to tell their story. This may give you some important information you can share with the doctor.
- The above conversation gives team members a chance to rave about their doctors.
- It's not only what you say that's important. How you say it and what you do can be more important. Talk in a comforting tone. Speak slower and softer than normal. Touch the patient appropriately as you speak and as the injection is given.
- If your team is great at handling patients with anxiety, mention this in your marketing materials. And describe the methods you use to alleviate anxiety.

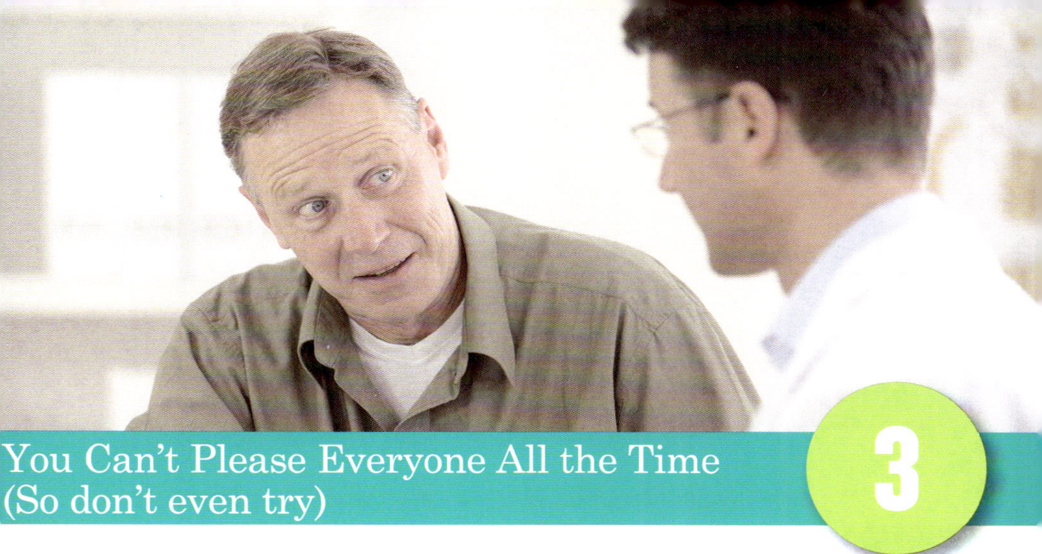

You Can't Please Everyone All the Time (So don't even try)

3

Whether it's in the dental office, the movie theater, or practically anywhere else, there's a contradiction in American culture. At once we espouse the notion of "one size fits all," but at the same time we recoil from it.

Why?

Because more often than not, one size does not fit all. And more importantly, you shouldn't even try. As the saying goes, you can't please all the people all the time. Sometimes, try as you might, it's better to turn down a prospective patient rather than sacrifice the dental practice ideals you've come to live by.

That doesn't mean giving up. It means honestly assessing whether or not a prospective patient is a good match for the type of dentistry you practice.

It takes courage, and yes, even a bit of humility. But walking away isn't a sign of defeat, nor is it arrogance. It's about having the confidence to chart your own dental course. Rather than trying to please everyone all the time, focus on pleasing some people as often as possible.

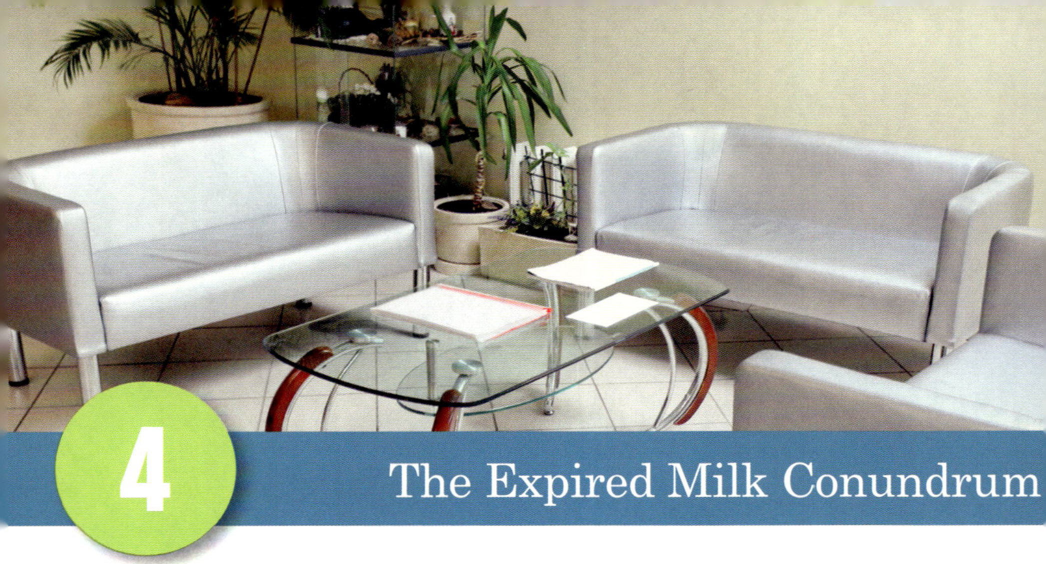

4 The Expired Milk Conundrum

Head to the supermarket milk aisle and what do you see? Rows and rows of milk with their expiration dates clearly marked.

Your goal as a consumer is simple: purchase the milk container with an expiration date furthest from the date you are shopping. Doing so (usually) ensures the freshest milk.

Dental practices face a similar challenge. While your products won't "spoil" in a bacterial sense, your offerings and how you market them, age with time. It's important to periodically review the products and services you're offering.

Ask yourself, are they the most innovative? Are they most in line with what your patients seek? Equally important: don't bury or hide older offerings with the newer material. Patients have a nose for such discrepancies – just like they do when they search for the freshest milk.

Don't fall into the trap of the expired milk conundrum!

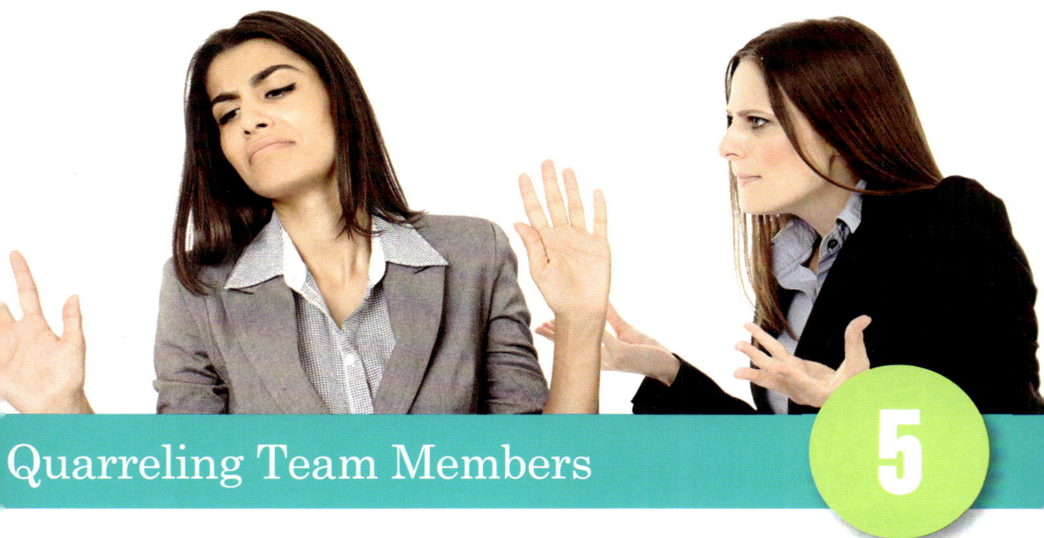

Quarreling Team Members

5

Whenever a group of people are confined in a relatively small space for extended periods of time, interpersonal conflicts will inevitably arise. When they do, you must take action quickly. Here is one way to do it if you have two team members who are quarreling... and it's been going on for a while. In a private setting, get the two people together, hand one of them $40 and say, "You two are going to lunch today on me. During lunch, work this out. It will be over when you return. If it's not, I will get involved. And trust me on this one. You don't want me to get involved."

This can't be a bluff. You must be willing to take immediate action including termination of one of the individuals. Prior to taking any disciplinary action, consult with your lawyer to be certain what you intend to do complies with your state's labor laws.

Don't sweep office problems under the rug. They love it in the darkness where they can grow and produce a flock of new, baby problems. Instead, shine a bright light on your office's interpersonal challenges. Face them. Solve them. And reap the benefits of a harmonious and successful practice.

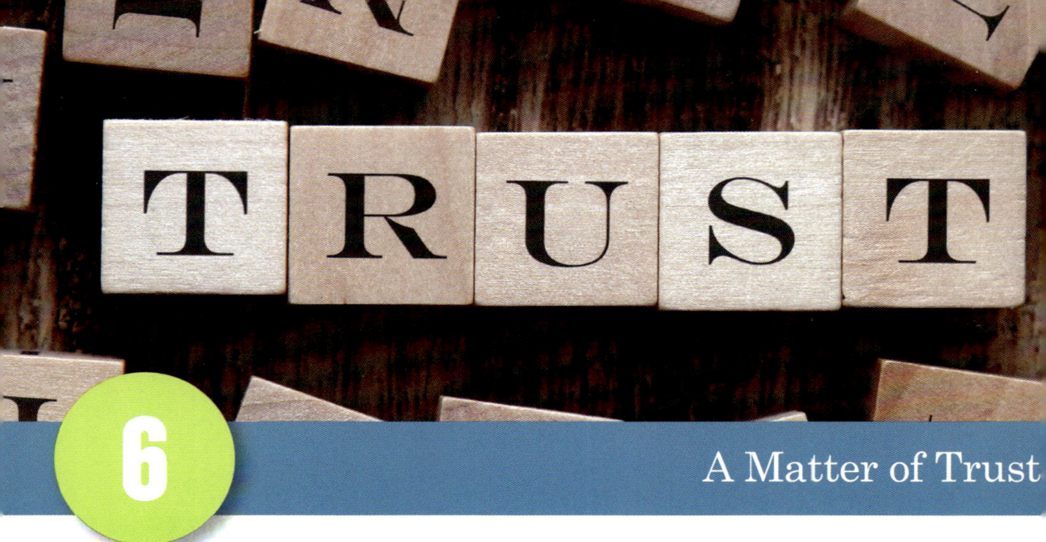

6 A Matter of Trust

Billy Joel had it right in his 1986 song. "It's always been a matter of trust."

For dentists tinkering in the human body's more delicate and intricate areas, trust is essential. And it trumps all other big marketing questions.

Whether it's worrying about specific product offerings, your social media outreach, or prices per procedure, nothing matters more than your ability to forge genuine connections with the people you treat.

If you've been in practice for several years and feel confident in your name recognition but haven't seen the level of customer conversions you expected, perhaps there is a trust issue that needs addressing.

Earning trust takes time. And it's difficult to measure. Your most loyal patients are likely to trust you more. Focus on engaging your newest patients to ensure that establishing trust is your top priority.

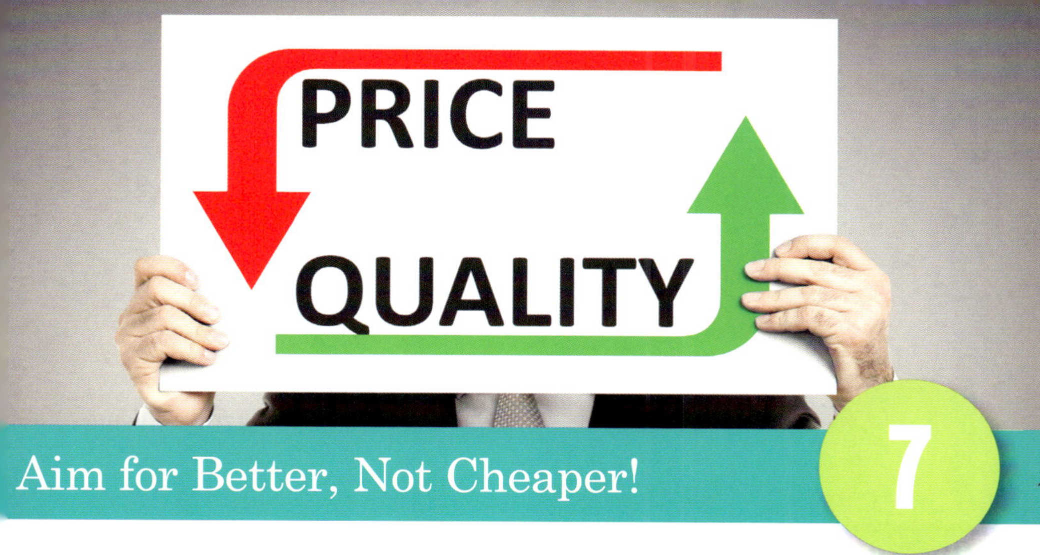

Aim for Better, Not Cheaper! 7

It's a kneejerk reaction common to many businesses: lower your prices to inspire a purchase.

Admittedly, it's a tactic that has economic merit. When stock prices drop low enough during daily trading, all of a sudden those stocks are purchased with breakneck speeds. Low prices encourage a buyer's market.

But when it comes to brick-and-mortar businesses like a dental office, the race to the price bottom should be cautioned against.

Rather than slashing prices, work to improve the quality of your product/s. Once your offerings have become that good they'll be difficult to ignore. Over time, patients will come to know you for the quality of your services and will care less about the cost of treatment.

Aim for better, not cheaper!

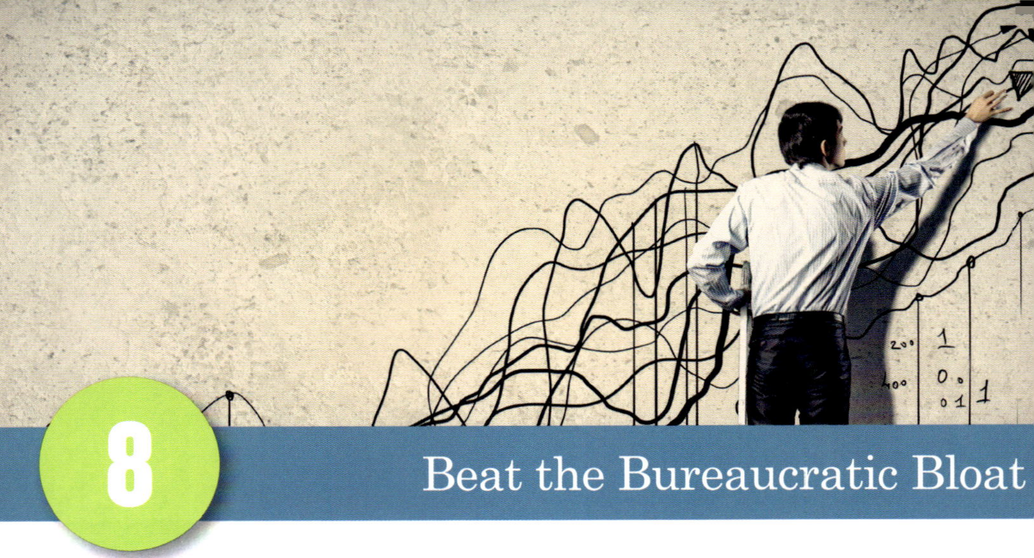

8 Beat the Bureaucratic Bloat

Just as physics has its set of immutable laws – what goes up must come down – organizations operate under their own logic.

A central tent of that logic is that as human and computer systems become more complex, the more failure prone they become.

It's not a hard concept to understand. Consider the US government and the degree to which bureaucracy undermines efficiency. Why? Because there are so many moving parts and self-interest dominates. Miscommunication and more importantly, misinterpretation, becomes increasingly common.

A dental office of a certain size (like any business) experiences these problems too. And like bureaucracies whose basic mission is one of self-preservation through risk averse behaviors, dental offices can also lose their dynamism.

Think about it. When you first became a dentist, chances are the profession inspired you, and you wanted to transform the lives of your patients. But over time, as the newness wore off, and new staff was added, a sense of complacency settled in.

Instead of being innovative, offering the latest treatments, augmented with cutting-edge imaging and in-house or outsourced milling, a dental practice weighed down by its own success starts to resist out-of-the-box thinking.

Like any large organization, self-preservation becomes key.

So how do you beat the bureaucratic bloat?

I'd tell you it's easy, but the truth is, it isn't. Recognizing your own institutional shortcomings is, however, a great first step. And it begins by taking a tip like this and using it as the springboard to schedule monthly or quarterly meetings. Ask the hard questions. Don't be afraid to challenge even your oldest, most loyal staff members to think differently.

It could even mean the temporary hiring of an executive coach to review your practice's performance. Whichever path you choose, don't give up! Keep fighting the good fight in the battle against bureaucratic BS.

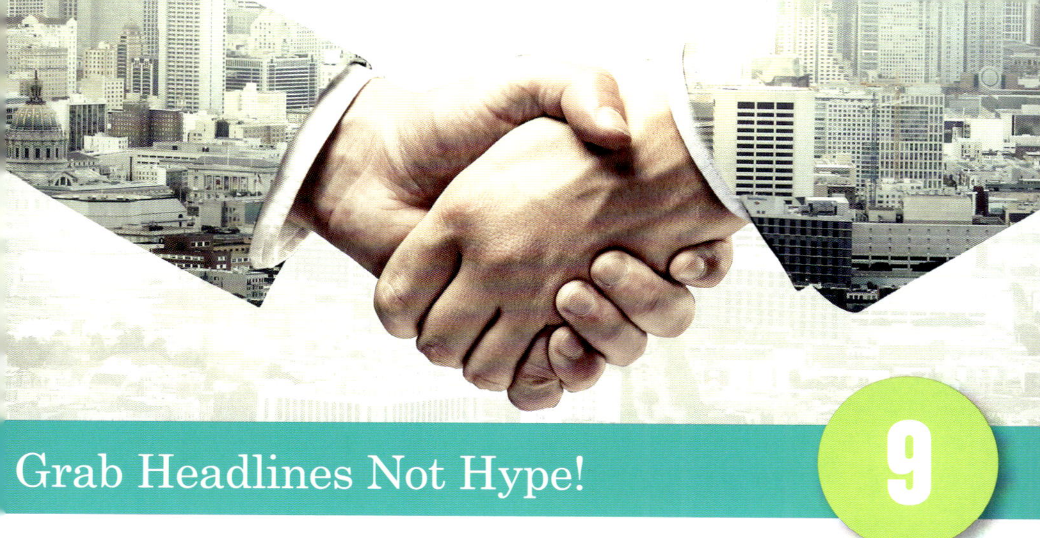

Grab Headlines Not Hype! 9

It's one of the most immutable marketing facts: sensationalism sells.

Whether it's over-the-top claims touting a new miracle drug, storm coverage on the local news, or a giant eyeball-grabbing billboard like the popular "Your Wife is Hot" signs on many U.S. roads, gaining people's attention is the name of the game.

But it's not the only game marketers must play. Very often when companies place too much emphasis on hype, they sacrifice honesty.

Dental practices are no different. While it's important to have diverse, multichannel patient engagement, it's equally important not to over promise and under deliver. Doing so erodes the most important quality you're trying to promote – trust.

Trust doesn't come package delivered and most of the time it can't be learned on the job. You have to earn it with every interaction, every procedure, and through every touch point. But over time, this intangible will factor prominently in a patient's decision to select your practice, and to continue selecting it for decades to come.

Once trust is firmly established and word-of-mouth marketing supports those efforts, you can re-up those headline grabbing efforts. Just keep the hype and hyperbole to a minimum and don't resort to sensational claims.

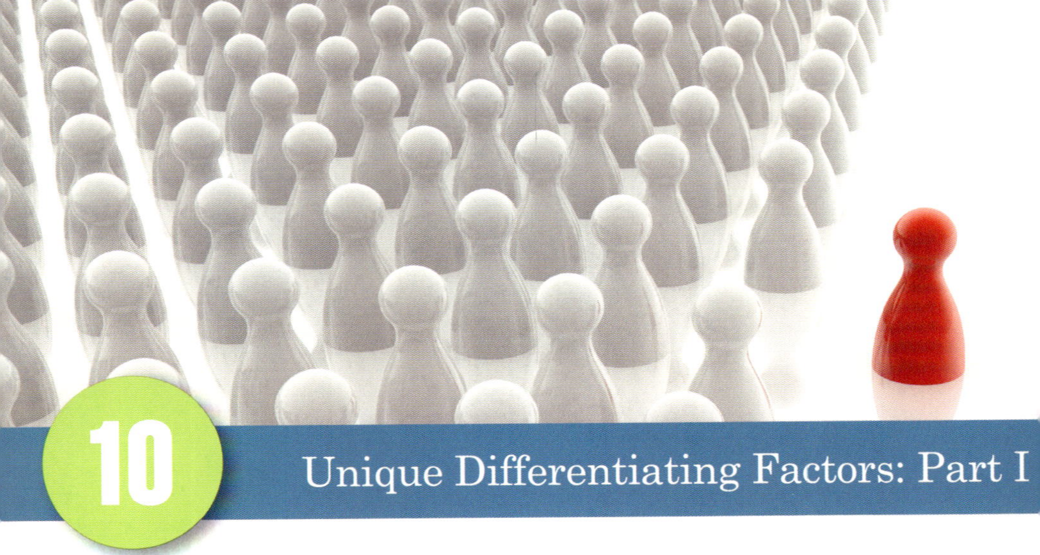

10 Unique Differentiating Factors: Part I

Answer the following questions:

- What makes your practice unique?
- What differentiates you from the competition?
- What would persuade a new patient to choose your practice even though you aren't listed as an in-network provider on her insurance plan?

In marketing terms, a UDF is your Unique Differentiating Factor. If you read 100 dentists' websites, office brochures or advertisements, you will quickly realize that they all send the same vanilla flavored messages such as:

- "We have a warm, friendly and caring team."
- "We take the time to get to know you."
- "We offer the finest dental care in the area."
- "We use the latest, cutting-edge technology."
- "We cater to all your dental needs."

Here's the acid test to determine if your UDF's are truly unique. If you called a random dental office and asked them, "Hey, do you guys have a warm, friendly and caring staff?" or "Do you guys take the time to get to know your patients?" Pretty much every office staff member would answer, "Yes" ... even if it really weren't entirely true. That means these statements are not really unique or differentiating.

Your UDFs must be noticeably different and compelling. To identify your UDFs, sit down with the team and brainstorm exactly what makes your office stand out from the crowd. How are you different in ways meaningful to patients? What benefits do you offer that patients really want? Benefits that are seldom offered by other offices in your area.

Be different in ways that people can see, appreciate and desire.

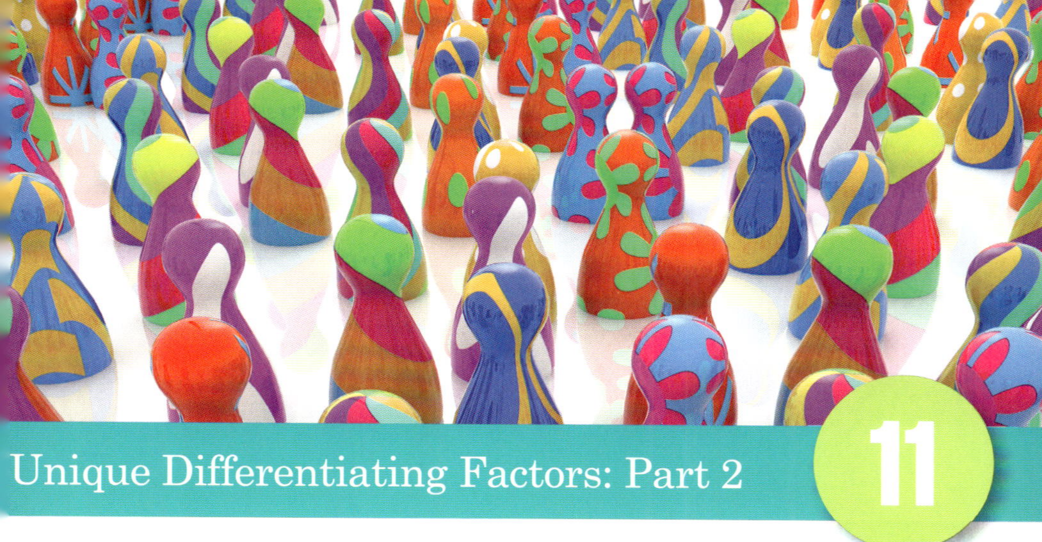

11 Unique Differentiating Factors: Part 2

Unique Differentiating Factors are the things that set you apart from other dentists. They are desirable factors that people can readily identify as being unique. Here are three of them:

Tired of Waiting for Your Dentist?

"Your time is as important and valuable as ours. We fully respect that. There's nothing more frustrating than rushing across town for your dental appointment and then sitting in somebody's office for 15 – 30 minutes after the agreed upon appointment time. In our office, if we say we will see you at 10 am, you will be seated within five minutes of your reserved time, your doctor or hygienist will be ready to see you and you will begin your care."

Do You Snore? Or Have You Been Diagnosed with Sleep Apnea?

"Snoring may be a sign of Obstructive Sleep Apnea which can have serious (in some cases life-threatening) consequences. Many patients with sleep apnea have been given CPAP machines, but can't tolerate them. If a physician or other health care practitioner certified in the diagnosis of sleep disorders has diagnosed Obstructive Sleep Apnea in a loved one or you, relief without the need for CPAP may be as close as our dental office. Dr. John Smith is trained and experienced in the use of oral devices for the treatment of Obstructive Sleep Apnea. Call for a consultation today."

Have a Denture that Won't Stay in Place?

Do you or anyone you know have a denture that won't stay put? If so, a "snap in" denture may be the answer. Local dentist, Dr. Maria Otis can help. She makes dentures that are retained by implants. The process is easier and quicker than you might imagine. See Dr. Otis to see if a "snap in" denture is right for you."

The above are three Unique Differentiating Factors that set a few, select offices apart and allow them to stand head and shoulders above the crowd. If you already have two or three unique differentiating factors, congratulations. To further set yourself apart, add another two or three factors that truly make you stand out. The public will notice. And you will benefit.

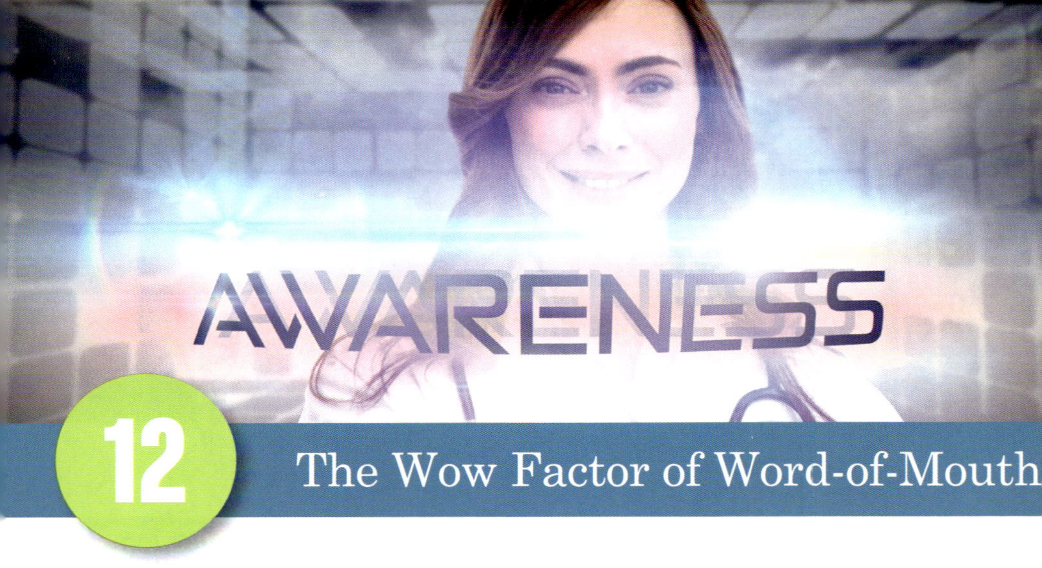

12 The Wow Factor of Word-of-Mouth

A bevy of technological innovation has businesses of all types and sizes racing to catch up in how they attract, retain and engage their customers.

Social media and digital interaction have driven much of this transformation. So whether you're a dentist, a hotelier, an amusement park operator, a corner hair salon, or any other establishment, these are exciting times to be living in.

But for all that's changed it's important to remember what hasn't: the power of word-of-mouth communication. Not just in terms of sharing Facebook posts, or Instagram pics, but in actual genuine human interaction.

We are, after all, a social species, intelligent mammals that gain significant information and social cues from direct real-world communication. Facetime and Skype and other digital outlets just don't cut it. It's not surprising, then, that according to communications firm Ogilvy, 74 percent of consumers still consider word-of-mouth as their key influencer for purchasing decisions.

Dental practices can use this old-school fact to their advantage. Encourage your patients to discuss their positive experiences with their friends and family. Perhaps even augment that effort by offering a promotional discount as they help recruit new patients. It doesn't have to be a large discount – something as little as 10 percent will do. That's enough to demonstrate good faith appreciation.

Word-of-mouth may seem a little dated. But it remains the most important tool in your dental practice patient recruitment.

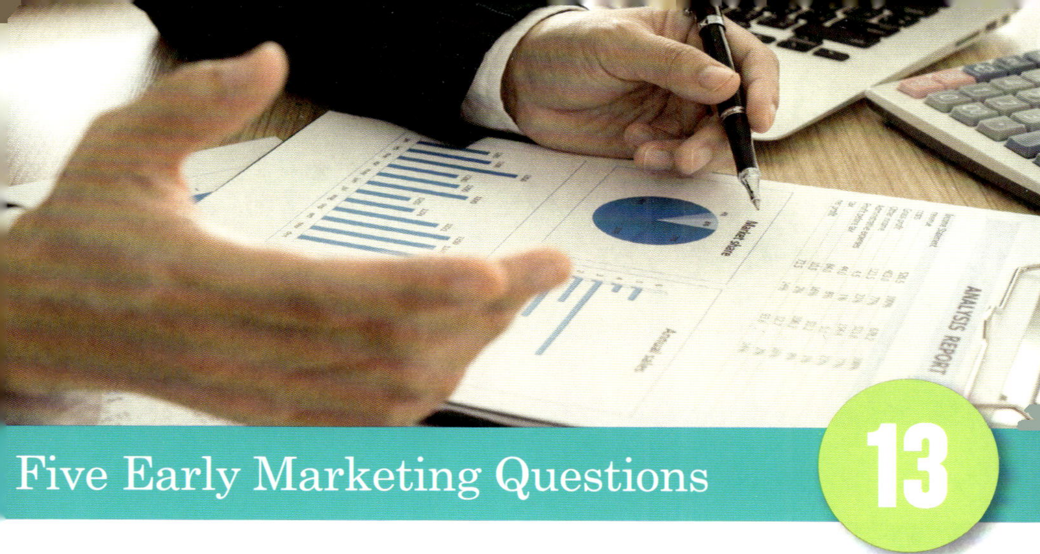

Five Early Marketing Questions 13

Before you spend a minute or a dollar on marketing, answer the following five questions:

1. Who, precisely, are you trying to reach?

If you're trying to reach everyone, you won't do an effective job of reaching anyone. What patient group or groups desire the kinds and quality of dentistry you want to provide?

2. What change are you trying to make?

Exactly, what do you want these people to do? Come to your office for a specialty service? Switch to your office from another one? Overcome their fears and see a dentist for the first time in years? Make their dental care more convenient with your location and office hours? If you don't know what change you want people to make, they won't know either.

3. How will you know if it's working?

Nineteenth century U.S. merchant, John Wannamaker, said, "Half the money I spend on advertising is wasted; the trouble is, I don't know which half." I know you've heard this a thousand times, but you must make the effort to track your marketing efforts.

4. How much time and money are you prepared to spend?

It seems like effective marketing always costs more than the plan said it would. What are your time and money limits? And do you have the fortitude to abide by these limits?

5. Who are you trying to please or impress?

I've seen several dental websites that look like they were designed to impress other dentists. Websites should be designed to make it easy for people to take the next step. Or to help a current patient learn more about your services and ask you about them. Or to influence a non-patient to pick up the phone and schedule an appointment.

It's less expensive to ask and answer these questions early than it is to spend time and money on the marketing later on.

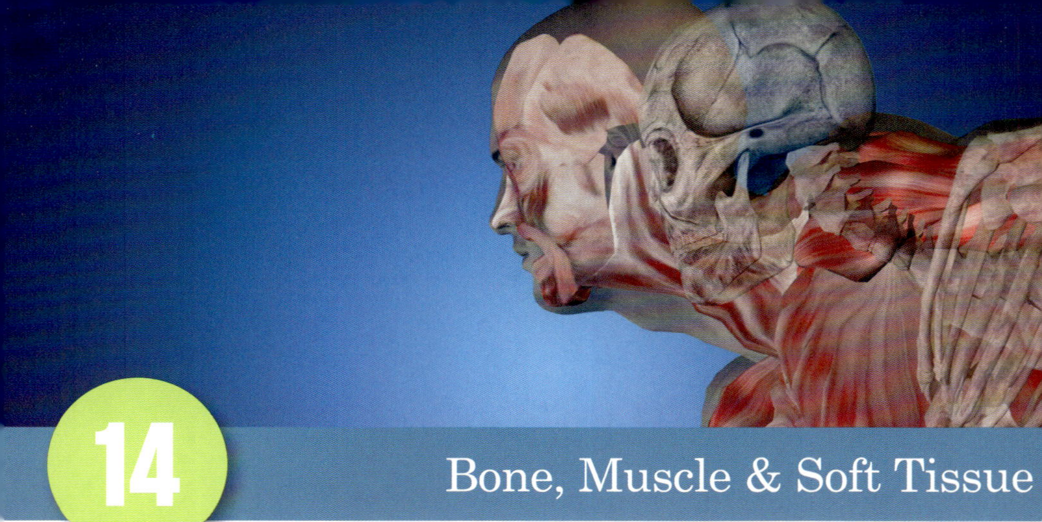

14 Bone, Muscle & Soft Tissue

Most dental teams are built with three types of people: Bone, Muscle & Soft Tissue.

Bone People are the skeletal framework. They exemplify your core values. The Bones have been around, have a mission and don't bend easily - even if no one is watching. The Bones say, "We don't do things that way around here."

Muscle People do the heavy lifting. They're the performers who can be counted on to do more than their share. And because they like to work, they do it without grumbling.

Soft Tissue People bring bulk which protects the muscles and the bones. The Soft Tissues can fill a room, handle details and add heft in many ways. They bring protection and cohesion. And sometimes they turn into muscle.

When Bone People break, you notice it. When those that make up your practice's skeleton leave or lose their ambition, the entire office gasps. And you often rush to fix the problem.

Muscle People are easily measured. You have many practice management tools to find and reward your best producers.

Soft tissue people are easy to add to your team, but harder to remove. They tend to bog down your practice with mediocre results and more management time.

A dental practice that lets itself be overwhelmed by too much soft tissue gets fat and happy. Then it stagnates or declines. The obvious answer to this unfortunate outcome is hire, train and retain the Bone and Muscle. And strategically trim the fat.

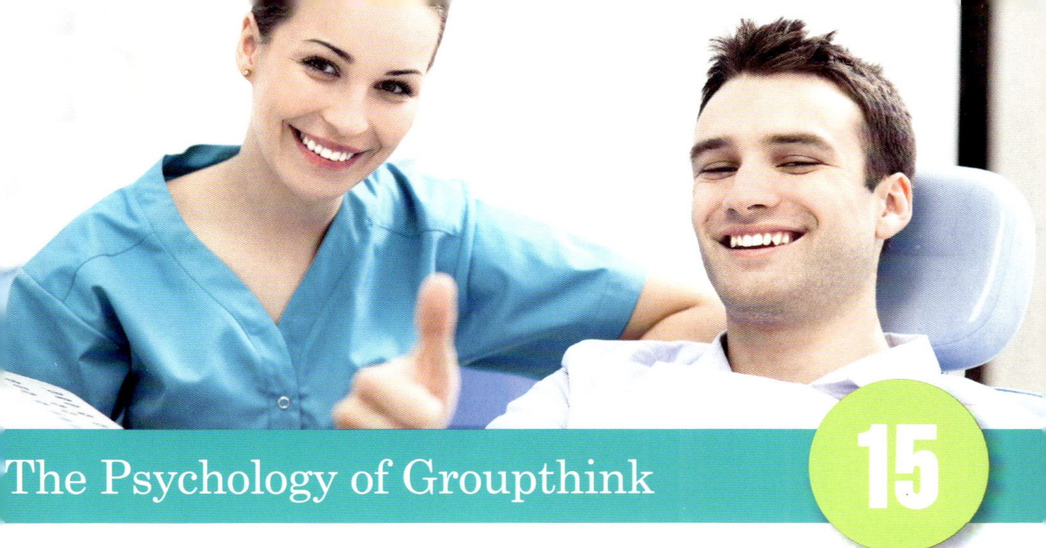

The Psychology of Groupthink

15

It's an experience to which we can all relate. Enjoy an expensive dinner at some fancy restaurant and invariably you're inclined to think the food was great – even if it wasn't.

The same logic applies in many situations: collective laughter at a comedy club, the satisfaction of a discount while shopping at an outlet store, etc. Situations elicit an expected reaction, even if reality doesn't match your expectations. We still laugh even when the joke isn't funny.

Let's face it; the dental office isn't a patient's favorite place to visit. Studies find that up to 80 percent of patients experience some anxiety just making the appointment.

If patients expect a less-than-pleasant experience, chances are they're going to get one. The key is to change the group think mentality. Aggressively promote your practice as delivering on the promise of a pain-free (or nearly pain-free) experience. It also helps if your front office staff goes out of its way to be kind, gentle and comforting – especially to the most anxious patients.

Over time, the group think will shift as patients expect – and help construct – their own positive experience.

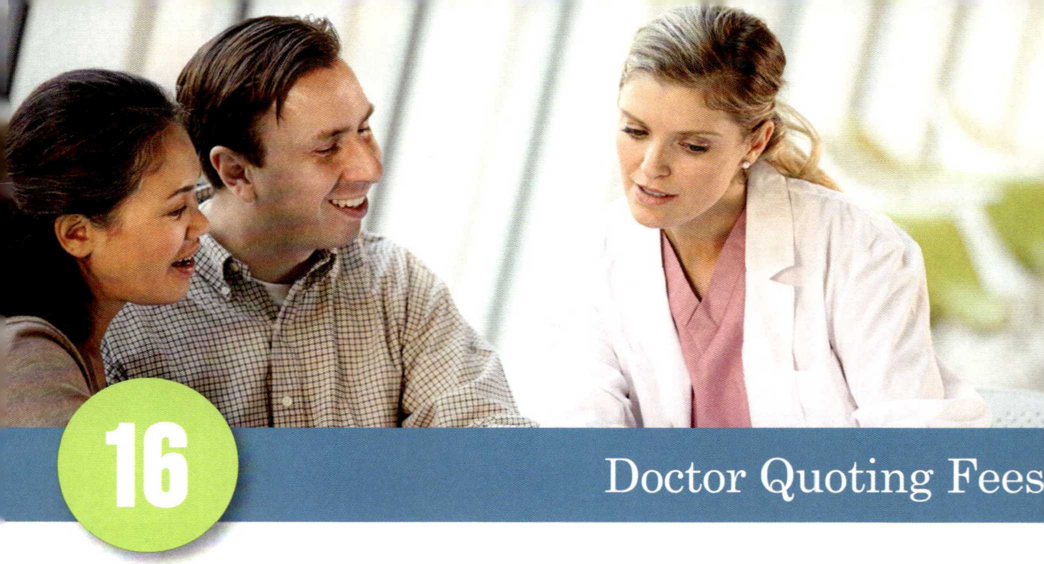

16 Doctor Quoting Fees

Many consultants teach that the doctor should never quote the fee. Leave that to your staff they say so you can be "professional." This advice is right in one respect, but wrong in another.

It's right in that some doctors routinely cave in to patients trying to bargain down the price. If you are guilty of this, stop it. You should decide who receives charity care. It's wrong in that for the most part patients have no clue how much their treatment may cost. And if you leave the room before they decide on the type of care they want, everyone loses.

Here's an example of what I mean. You advise a Mrs. Johnson to remove four, large, failing amalgams. She seems to understand the need for care and the reasoning behind placing build-ups and crowns. It seems like she is on the same page with you. But if you walk out of the room without discussing fees, you increase your risk of her doing nothing.

You left Mrs. Johnson feeling that she would move forward with the recommended care. When she gets to the front desk and sits down with your financial coordinator, she discovers the recommended care will cost several thousand dollars out of pocket. By this time, you're involved in another procedure. So she asks your financial coordinator, "I need to get this done, but I didn't know it would be that expensive. Isn't there something else we can do?" That's a question only you can answer.

I don't recommend you quoting the exact fee or getting involved in working out the method of payment. That should be left to your financial coordinator. Here's what I recommend saying: "Mrs. Johnson, I can't give you an exact fee at this point or what your insurance will cover. Maria will do that for you at the front desk. However I can give you an approximate figure. The care we discussed will be somewhere between $4,000 and $4,400. I'm sure Maria will work out something that's comfortable for you."

There are two ways Mrs. Johnson may respond:

She breathes heavily, but realizes the importance of receiving the best dental care. She thanks you and agrees to have the care done.

She breathes heavily and says, "I had no idea it was going to be that expensive. Is there something else we can do?"

Now you have a chance to discuss other options. What treatment you present depends upon the patient's needs and your philosophy of care. Now, you can help Mrs. Johnson move forward with your first plan or an alternative one.

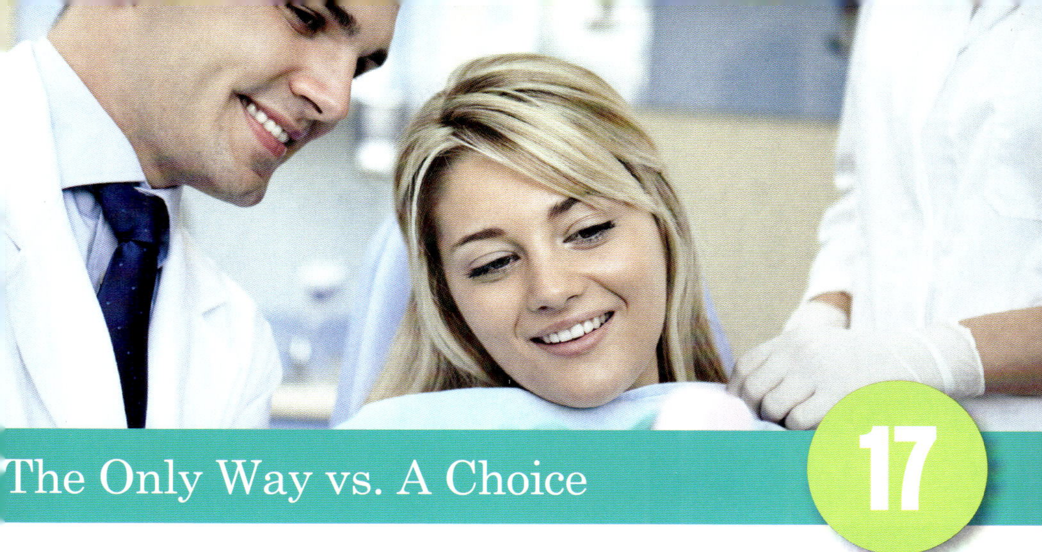

17 The Only Way vs. A Choice

Most of us react poorly to being told, "This is the only way you can do it." In response, we tend to think, "Oh, yeah!" Or, even worse, "Based on what I know, I don't think you're right!" Our instinct is to respond to "The Only Way" with confrontation. We react emotionally instead of responding intelligently.

I see this happening all the time in dental offices. As an example, when a tooth is missing, the dentist says, "You should place an implant in that space." In effect, the dentist is saying, "This is the only way."

Unless patients mention that they desire implants, give them a choice by saying, "Given your situation, you have several choices:

- "You can do nothing. The problems with that choice are …"
- "You can have a removable partial denture made. The problems with that choice are ..."
- "You can have a fixed bridge placed. The problems with that choice are …"
- "You can have an implant placed. The advantages of that choice are …"

Giving your patients choice between two or more forms of dental care is a generous act. It's a form of truth telling that benefits them and you. All choices have consequences. Helping patients understand them in advance leads to better decisions on their part and higher case acceptance rates of the best options on your part.

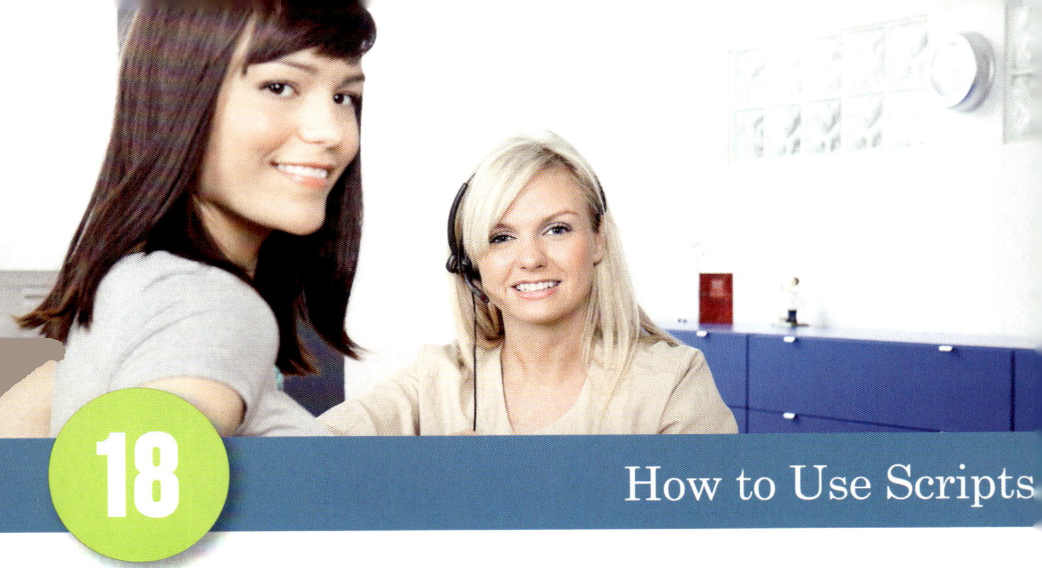

18 How to Use Scripts

I think scripts are great. But for the scripts to have real power, the user must own the words. If you ask someone to use a script they don't believe in or that doesn't feel comfortable to them, you're shooting them (and yourself) in the foot. They either won't use the script because it's too painful to do so, or they'll use the script, but betray the message by the incongruency of their voice qualities and body language.

So, when you want your team to use scripts, give them a sample script using the words you believe are best. Then have people rewrite the scripts in their own words while retaining the full meaning of the script you provided. Then have your team members practice their scripts until the words naturally roll out of their mouths. Now their words, voice qualities and body language will match. They will be congruent, and the message will be communicated effectively.

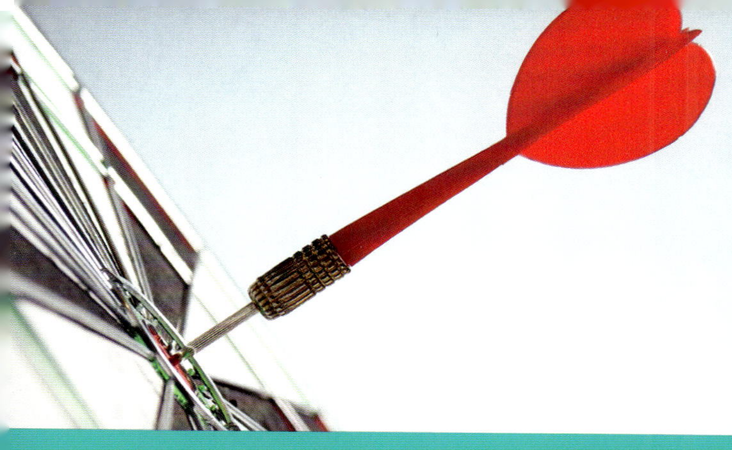

Game On for the Long Game! 19

If you're a dental practice just starting out, it's likely you can expect decades in the business. Way to go!

While it would be great to have a crystal ball, to predict with perfect accuracy what's to come, it's an unrealistic scenario. Accuracy, or your powers of prediction, is only as accurate as the information you have at hand. Can you get lucky and guess the next trend? Sure. Luckier still is if you're that innovator who can drive the next change – before the dental industry or your patients even know they need it. This is what the late Steve Jobs was known for.

Short of being the next Steve Jobs, a better strategy can be distilled from two expressions that come to us from the financial services industry – "hedge your bets" and "diversify your portfolio."

Both terms relate to managing risk. Lacking complete predictive powers it's better to plan a practice management strategy that is goal setting, but flexible. You must be able to adapt quickly to changes in regional, local, and national economic and dental trends should the need suddenly arise.

It helps to act like a palm tree. Under the right growing conditions, coconut palms can live up to 90 years. Their ability to bend with the wind is a key strategy for their longevity. When your dental practice bends to the winds of change you can be sure you'll enjoy many years of successful practice.

Denial is another "strategy" to watch out for. In a dental practice denial manifests more like complacency – a refusal to accept that times are changing. Instead of quick thinking and adaptability, the dental practice in denial does things the way they've always been because that's just the way it is.

Remember, whether you're a new practice just starting out, or a veteran of the dental industry, keep the long game in mind and you can expect a lifetime of professional success.

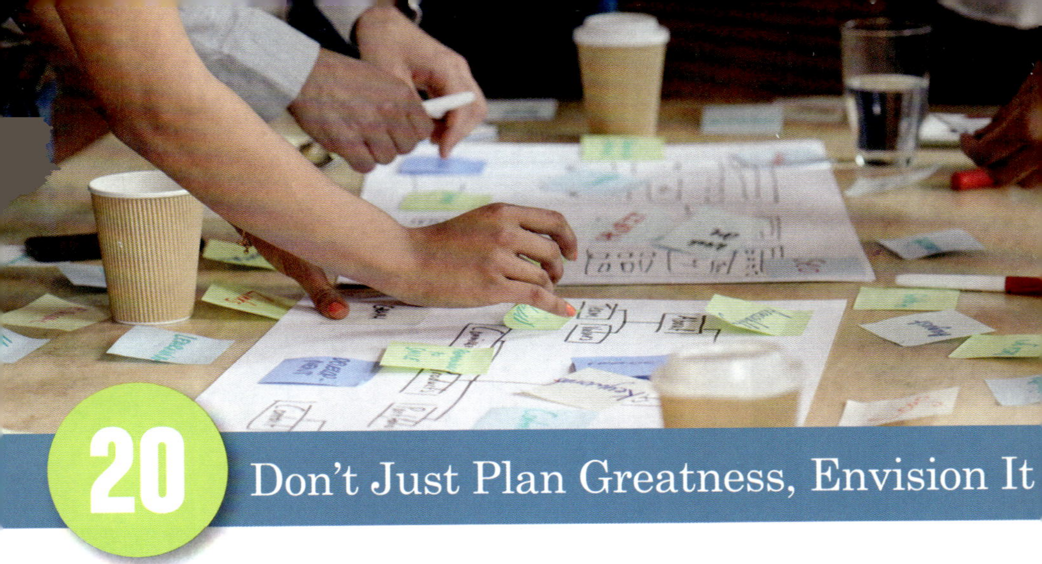

20 Don't Just Plan Greatness, Envision It

Many tips in this book attempt to steer the reader toward concrete action, or they offer new insights into how to improve your dental practice business model.

But sometimes its important to put down the pen and paper (or tablet and keyboard) and take a different approach. Executing dental practice success begins with first envisioning it.

What does that mean? It means taking the time to imagine what success looks like for you. Sure, take some time and write these thoughts down. But don't turn the mental exercise into a rigorous test. Freeform thinking is a way to inspire your entire staff. Have fun with it. Bounce ideas off each other, and don't be afraid to dream big!

The key is to make the process interactive. Perhaps schedule a meeting over a long lunch (possibly catered). Plan this well in advance so that there are no disruptions with phone calls or patients. Consider a day on the calendar where you know it will be quiet. Pair up colleagues in teams to brainstorm the best ideas.

Topics to consider may include:

- How to better engage patients
- What new incentives or offers could you provide?
- How else can you connect with and integrate with the community at large?
- What new procedures would you like to incorporate in the next six months?
- How else can you make the employee experience more efficient, but also more rewarding?

These are just some of the ideas you should consider. Before long, with meetings that encourage this type of thinking, your dental practice dreams will transform into dental practice reality!

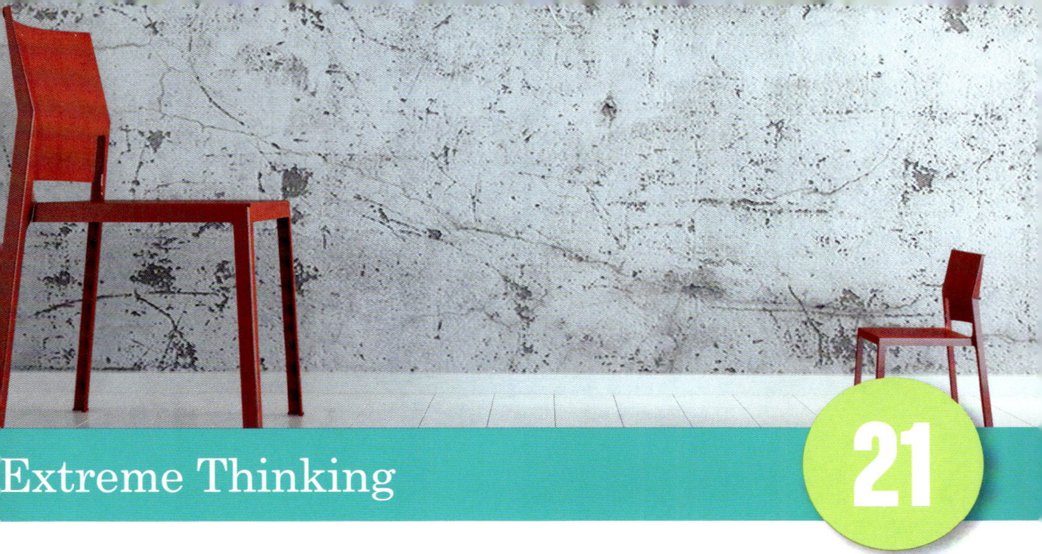

Extreme Thinking

21

You could build a dental practice dedicated to paying your team members ever more. Or you could build a practice based on paying them ever less.

You could create a dental practice based on the idea of charging your patients the lowest possible fees. Or you could charge fees that are in the top 5%.

You could offer the best care that dentistry has to offer. Or you could just present treatment plans you believe patients will accept.

It's tempting to view each of these extremes as an alternative to compromise. But compromise isn't a goal, it's a temporary tactic. The real question is, "Where are you headed, and which options will best get you there?"

To move your practice forward, you must push against the status quo and make difficult choices. The closer these choices are to the extremes (on one end or the other), the harder they are to make.... which is exactly why most dentists don't like to make them. And they quickly compromise to maintain their comfort levels.

So what are a few extreme choices that are best for you? Time to choose.

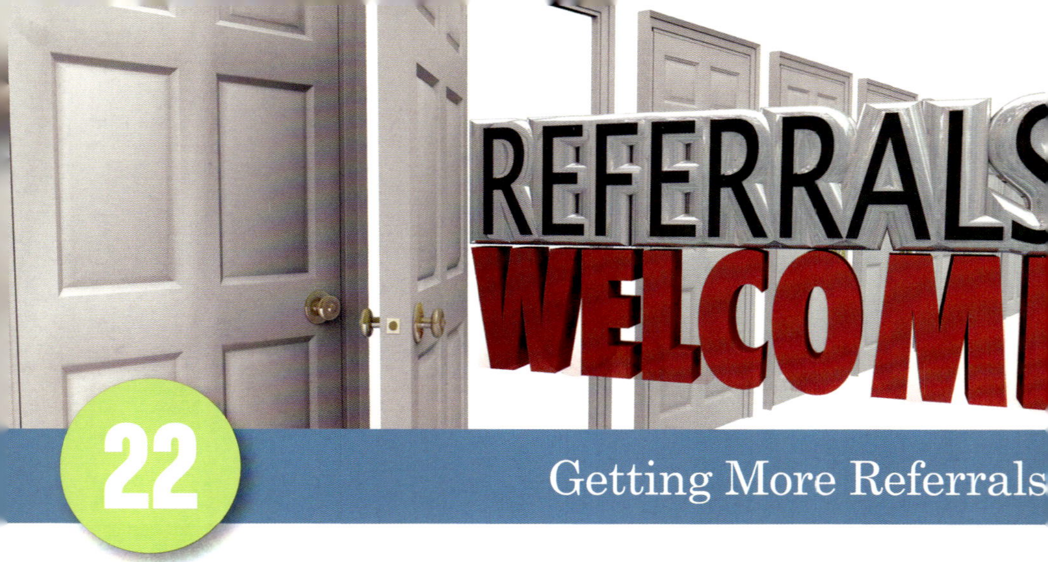

22 Getting More Referrals

Because birds of a feather tend to flock together, referrals to your practice from your existing patients tend to be the best new patients. Here are two tips to help you get more of them.

Tip #1 - Focus on Referrals from Your New Patients.

Most dentists assume the patients who are most likely to refer are those who have been with them the longest. This is not the case. New patients are two times more likely to refer patients to you. So say to your new patients at their final visit of the series, "We hope you enjoyed your experience with us." They will almost always answer in the affirmative.

Then ask, "Could you help us help another patient?" They will say, "Sure." Then say, "I'd really appreciate your help in telling somebody else about our office. Would you be willing to give two of these referral cards to your family, friends, coworkers or a new neighbor?" Giving them very specific places to think about will help them picture exactly who they can refer to your practice.

Tip #2 - Ask Them When They're at a Moment of High Reciprocity.

Influence expert, Dr. Robert Cialdini, teaches that people are most likely to respond favorably to a request right after they express their appreciation for something you did for them. As an example, Mr. Sahabi says, "I can't believe that you already gave me the injection. I didn't feel a thing!"

You reply, "Mr. Sahabi, I'm thrilled for you. You're a terrific patient. Could you help me help another patient?" One hundred percent of the time he will ask how he can help. When he does agree, say, "I'd really appreciate your help in telling somebody else about our office. Would you be willing to give two of these referral cards to your family, friends, coworkers or a new neighbor?"

Don't passively wait for referrals to happen. Create a specific plan and team reward system to actively create referrals.

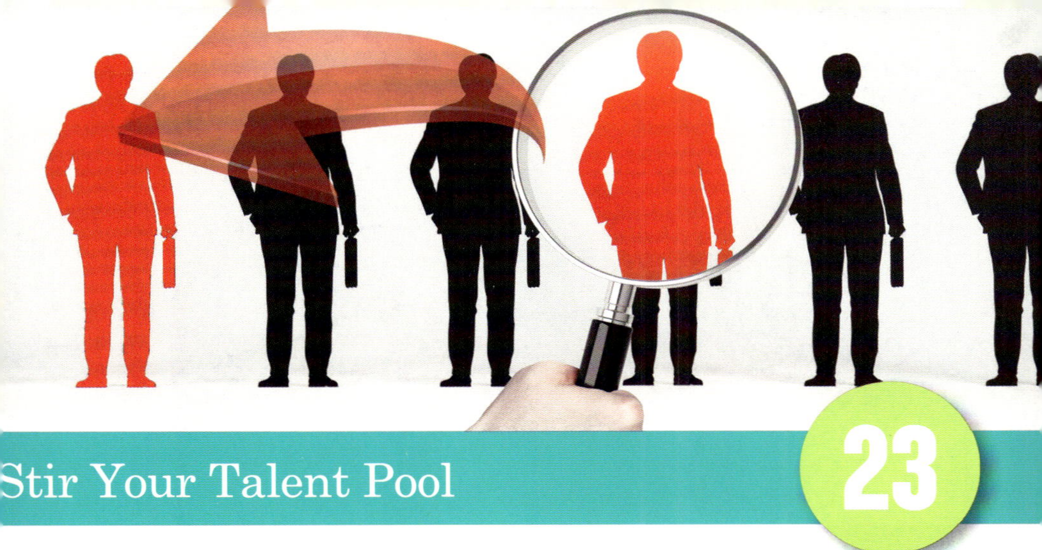

Stir Your Talent Pool

23

When you work in a dental practice, it's easy to think of your staff members as fitting a specific job title. After all, that s what they were hired for.

But remember each individual is much more han his or her title alone. Think of your team as a talent pool. And just because someone is currently engaged in a particular role, doesn't mean they can't learn new skills or try out new roles – even on a rotating basis.

Newsrooms operate under a similar principle. Reporters all possess a related skill. They can write and report the news, although their beats – their subjects of focus – vary. While t's great to have your best writers covering the topics they are most comfortable with, some editors like to mix it up a bit. Every few months reporters shift beats.

The result of such effort is obvious: reporters earn new material, cultivate new sources of nformation, and generally see their new beat n a different light than their colleague – if for no other reason that it's human nature. No two people see the same thing alike.

To be sure, mixing up talent in a dental office can be tricky. Not all of your staff has identical skills. But, within the natural confines of our profession, it might help if you rotate positions from time to time – especially positions that relate to front office management and patient care.

The benefits of this exercise might be difficult to measure at first. But over time, it's likely your office morale will improve, renewed interest will be encouraged, and a positive working atmosphere will permeate the office.

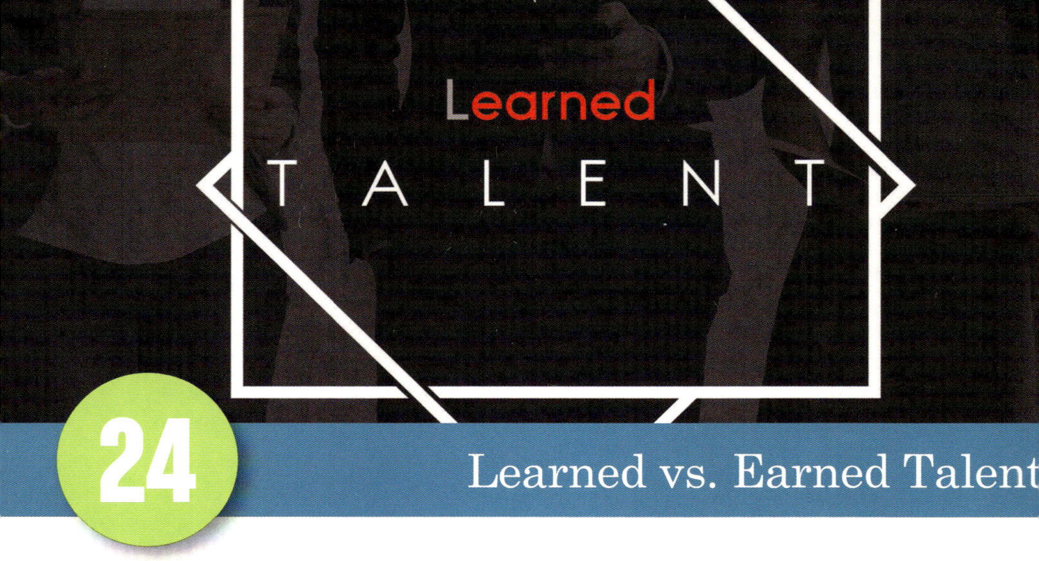

24 Learned vs. Earned Talent

From my experience as a dental practice owner and national lecturer, I've come to recognize two types of talent. I call them "learned" vs. "earned" talent. And increasingly, I find that business leaders confuse their meaning – even if they call these talents by different names.

So what is learned talent and what is earned talent?

Learned talent speaks to character attributes many of us aspire to possess. Some of the most common include:

- Honesty
- Thoughtfulness
- Generosity
- Positive
- Likability
- Proactive
- Flexibility
- Fun

The trouble is, too often people think these attributes are earned by birthright or upbringing, when in fact they can be learned!

Earned talent is much more selective. Some people inherit superior math or communication skills. Some people are innately better runners, etc. etc. The talent in these scenarios is "earned" to the extent that people are born with it.

But the exciting fact is that so much of what you look for in dental office chemistry can be learned! Consider that the next time you notice a colleague slacking!

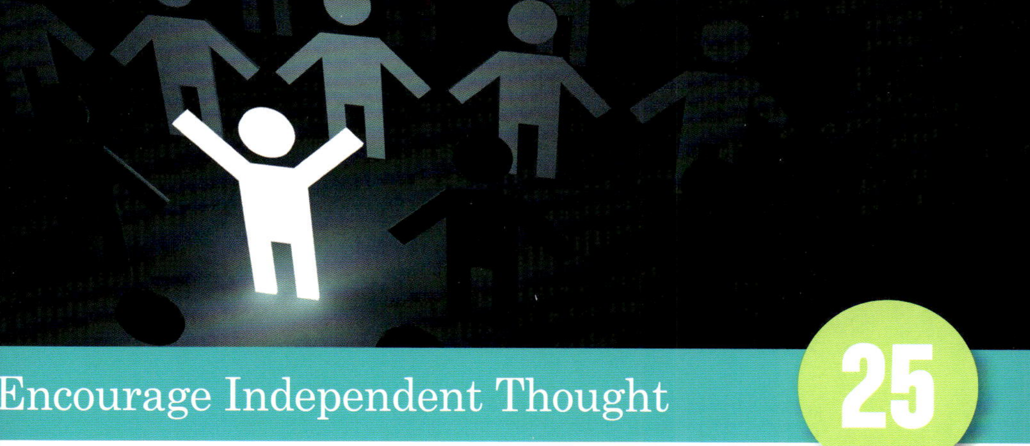

Encourage Independent Thought

25

In today's office a balance of leadership style is constantly being played out: the balance between authority and independent thinking.

Traditionally this wasn't always the case. Especially in industrial and/or military settings independent thought can cripple an operation. Imagine if an assembly line worker decided to install a key car component "just the way he or she liked to." Failure to adhere to industrial standards could result in fatal injury or lost millions in recalled parts.

Your dental office requires both a steady hand and flexibility. Of course, dental implants and complicated surgeries need to be performed to exacting specs.

But when it comes to patient interaction and front office management, make sure that you seek the advice of the men and women working "in the trenches." Chances are they are extremely knowledgeable about what your patients require and the types of treatment they need. Don't be afraid to encourage employees to speak their mind in a professional manner.

That encouragement will build employee confidence, tends to enhance their feelings of self-worth, and ultimately will make for a better worker.

So be sure to encourage independent thought if you want to take your dental practice to the next level!

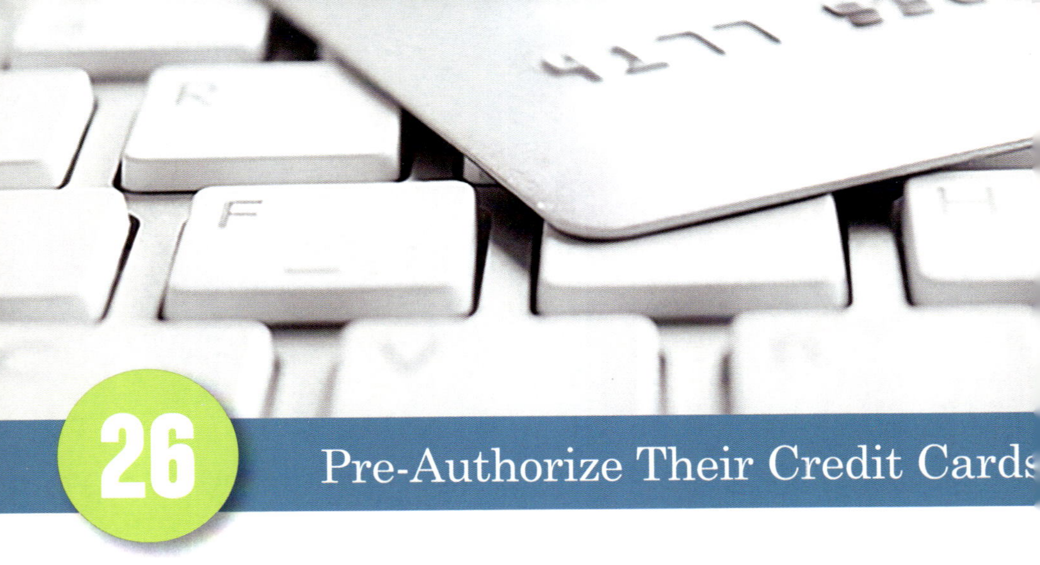

26 Pre-Authorize Their Credit Cards

An excellent strategy to receive payment at the time of treatment is to pre-authorize the use of your patients' credit cards for unpaid balances after receipt of insurance payment. Here is a sample script with comments.

Team Member: "For your convenience, we can pre-authorize your credit card. After we receive payment from your insurance company, the card will be automatically run to take care of any balance due."

Patient: "Why do I need to do that? My insurance pays for everything."

Team Member: "It is possible that your insurance will pay for 100% of your care at each visit. If that's the case, no charge will be made to your card. However, most insurance companies only pay 100% of their allowable fee which are probably less than our fees. If this is the case, we will process the unpaid balance with your card. This will save you time and hassle."

Patient: "I don't like leaving my card information with anyone."

Team Member: "I understand your concern. Just as you trust us with the confidentiality of your medical records, you can trust us with this information."

Patient: "Just send me a bill after my insurance company pays."

Team Member: "To keep your costs down, we've eliminated billing. We don't want to raise our fees to cover billing expenses."

Money conversations can be challenging, especially if your team members are winging it and don't have a script. That's why scripting and role-playing are vital to your practice's success.

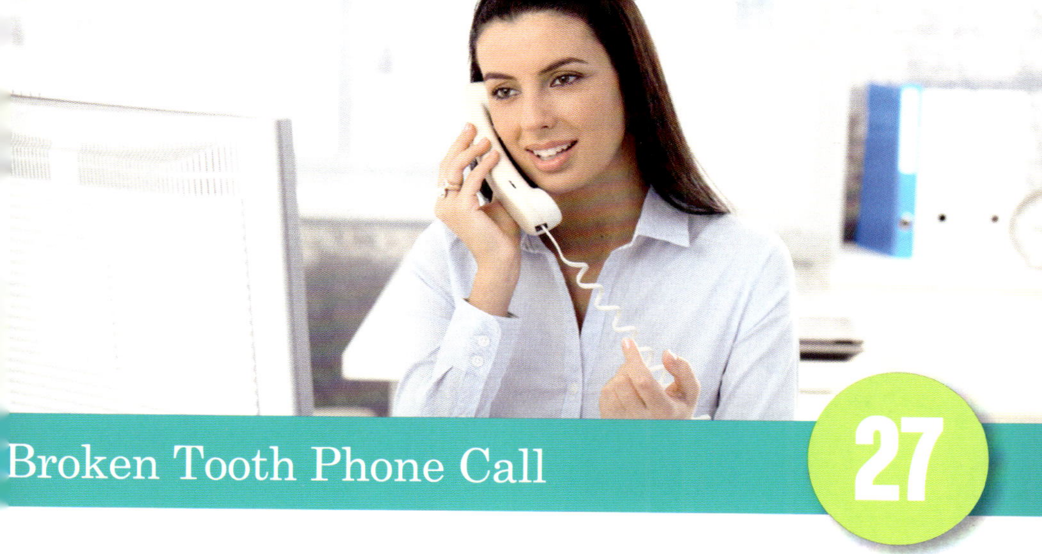

Broken Tooth Phone Call

27

Let's discuss the Broken Tooth Phone Call. I will give you a sample script and then discuss the process.

Patient: "Hi, this is Marilyn Clark. I broke a back tooth this morning. Can I get in today to see the doctor?"

Team Member: "I'm happy to help you Ms. Clark. Do you have any discomfort?"

Patient: "It's real sharp and irritating my tongue."

Team Member: "I understand. I will make sure we get you in today. When was your last visit with us?"

Patient: "I've never been to your office before."

Team Member: "Okay, how does 3pm sound?"

Patient: "Sounds great."

Team Member: "We'll see you as quickly as possible, but there may be a short wait today. Do you need directions to our office?"

Patient: "I know right where you are."

Team Member: "Excellent. In order for the doctor to help you today, he will need to do an examination and take an x-ray. The exam is $40 and the x-ray is $25. You can take care of that today with cash, check or credit card before you leave the office. Will that work for you?"

Patient: "That's fine."

Team Member: "Ms. Clark, we may need to have you come back for more care, but the doctor will do everything possible to make you comfortable today. I look forward to seeing you at 3."

Call Discussion

- After you learn it, use the caller's name during the conversation.
- If the patient is having discomfort, see the patient the same day.
- If they may have to wait in the reception area, tell them that.
- Make sure the patient knows where your office is.
- Tell them the fees will be due at the time of service. If you don't, they may think nothing is due.

Role-play the above conversation with all team members who answer the phone.

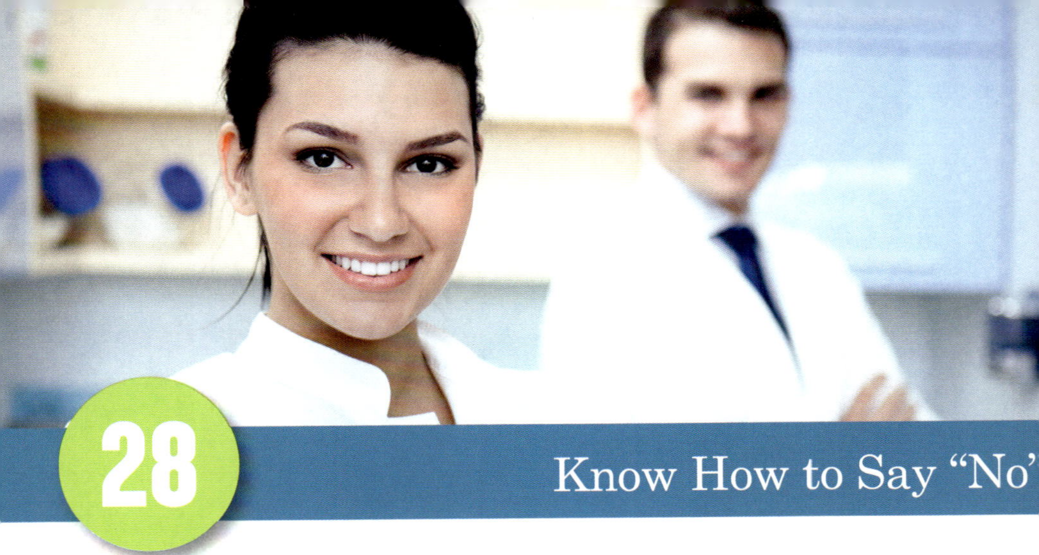

28 Know How to Say "No"

It's amazing how difficult such a small two-letter word can be to say. That's especially true if you're what psychologists call a "people pleaser."

While it's good to be a people pleaser some of the time, at other times people pleasers run the risk of trying too hard; of doing too much for other people and not believing in their own self worth.

In a dental practice, it might seem like the most natural thing in the world to "yes" your patients to the hilt.

But if your practice really doesn't offer what they seek, it's perfectly appropriate to let patients down gently. Have the confidence to say 'no' while offering those potential patients helpful advice as they seek a better professional fit.

Sometimes professional integrity starts with saying 'No.'

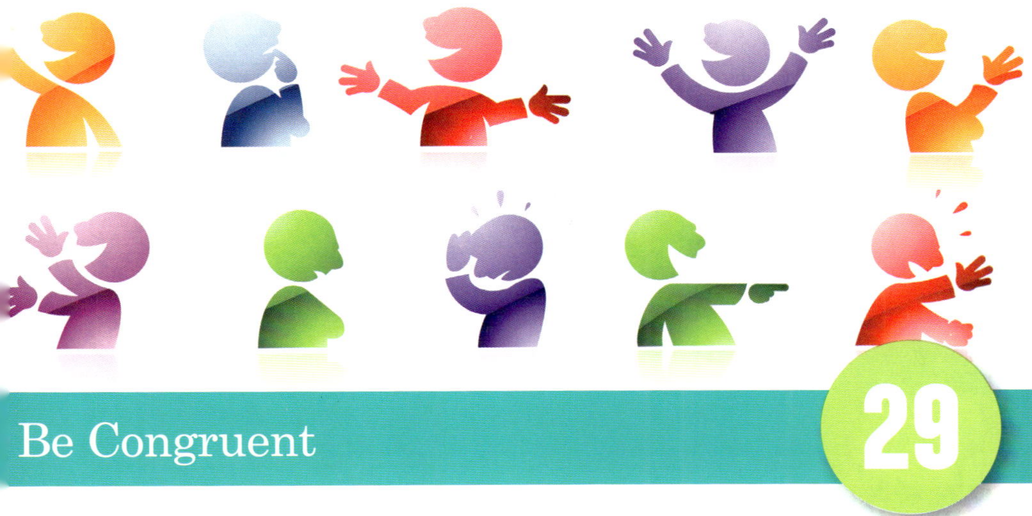

Be Congruent

29

When you're incongruent, your words say one thing and your voice qualities and/or body language say the opposite. Here's an example. Your dental supply person's words say, "Those supplies will definitely be in your office next Tuesday." But their voice qualities and body language are saying, "I'm not so sure about that."

When you're congruent, your words, voice qualities and body language all send the same message. When a congruent message is heard, people think, "This person really believes what they're saying." And they will take your message to heart and act on it in a positive way.

Belief is the key to congruency. People who believe in something will automatically use the words, voice qualities and body language that all head in the same direction. I see this happening all the time with our Implant Seminars students. They come to us unsure in their ability to place and restore implants. But with the acquisition of knowledge and practical, hands-on experience, their belief grows. And after placing their first few implants, their belief blossoms. Now they believe, their teams believe and their patients believe. Belief is contagious, and your congruency is the carrier. Harness its power whenever you communicate.

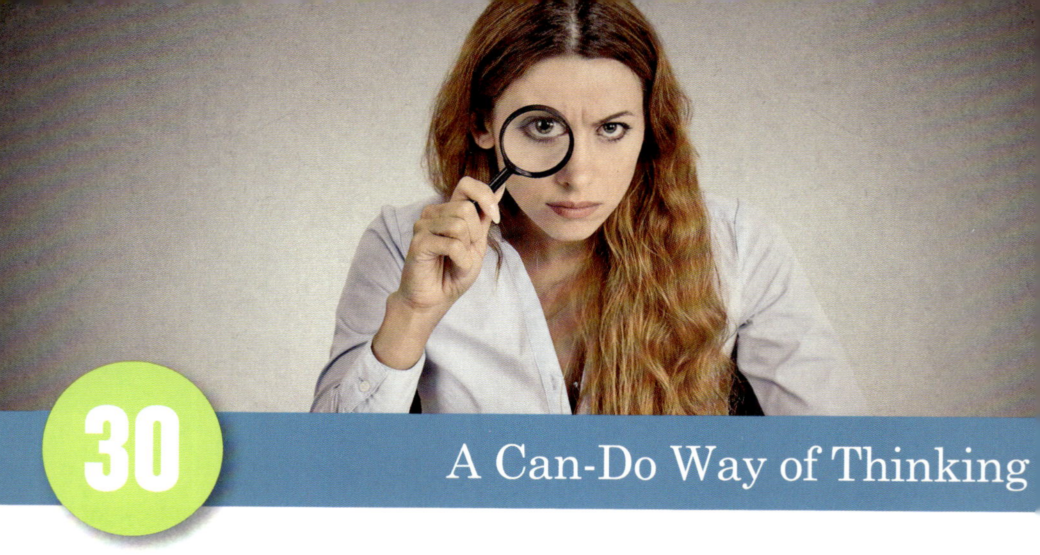

30 A Can-Do Way of Thinking

Staying positive all the time under all circumstances is unrealistic at best and downright harmful at worst.

But if your dental practice is looking to recruit new staff it's better to err on the side of can-do thinkers.

Can-do thinkers aren't afraid to dream big and they aren't afraid to fail. And they're certainly not afraid to speak their mind.

Naysayers envision themselves as a lonely voice of reason in an irrational sea of anything is possible. But the truth is, very often these people are selfish. They are selfish because their caution is typically rooted in the risks that a given venture poses to them and not the company at hand.

A can-do thinker should be easy to recognize in the interview process. Seek them out. As for your existing staff, if you suspect a cannot-do thinker, sit them down for an informal, but important meeting. Constructive attitudes go a lot further in the dental office than destructive attitudes and that this is something that needs to be worked on.

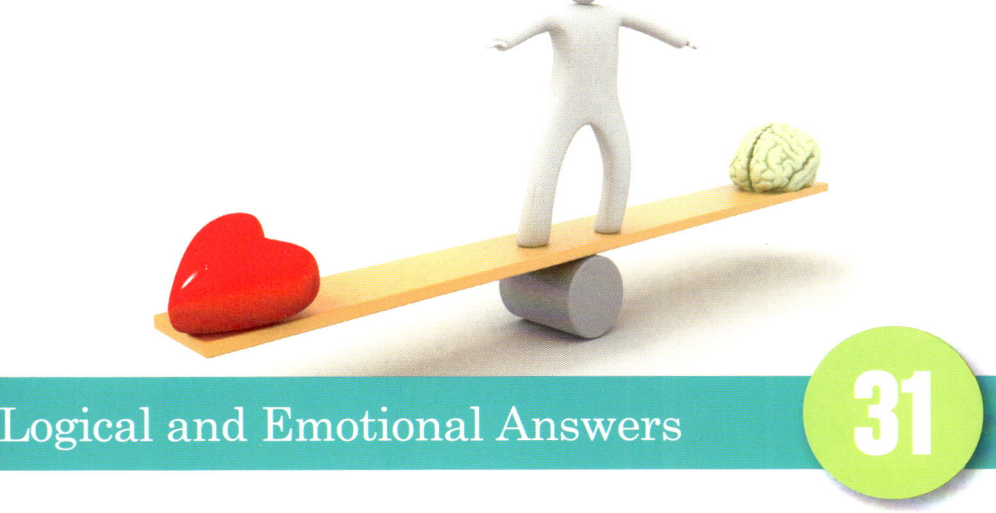

Logical and Emotional Answers

31

In your office, people ask you questions and bring up concerns all the time. How you respond to them is an important component of the trust and rapport you establish. Some of these questions and concerns are logical. Logical questions and concerns in dentistry usually address materials and procedures. Respond to the logical questions and concerns with logical responses.

Some questions and concerns are emotional. Respond to these with emotional responses. Emotional questions and concerns typically address fear, pain, money, time and appearance.

Being logical creatures, we dentists tend to respond to all of these questions and concerns with logical responses. Here's an example:

Patient – "I'm really afraid of having all those implants done."

Dentist – "There is no need to worry, Tom. We will sedate you with Diazepam and use a local anesthetic. You will be fine."

You logically answered his question, but does Tom really feel any better after hearing your response? I don't think so. "Feel" is the key word in the previous sentence. Here's another way to answer the concern with the Feel, Felt, Found Formula:

Patient – "I'm really afraid of having all those implants done."

Dentist – "I totally understand how you feel, Tom. We had a guy in here last month who felt the same way. After his implants were completed, he found that it was way easier than he imagined. We will take great care of you and make sure that you are as comfortable as possible through the entire process."

Here is a three-step exercise that will improve the case acceptance of your comprehensive dentistry:

1. Make a list of the Top Ten Tough Questions and Concerns you hear that are related to comprehensive dentistry.
2. Make another list of patients who had similar questions and concerns, completed their treatment and were happy they did.
3. Match lists 1. and 2. above to create 10 Feel, Felt, Found responses. Then role-play your responses several times until they easily flow out of your mouth.

Be flexible. Learn to respond logically and emotionally when the situation demands. Your patients will feel better, and you will do better.

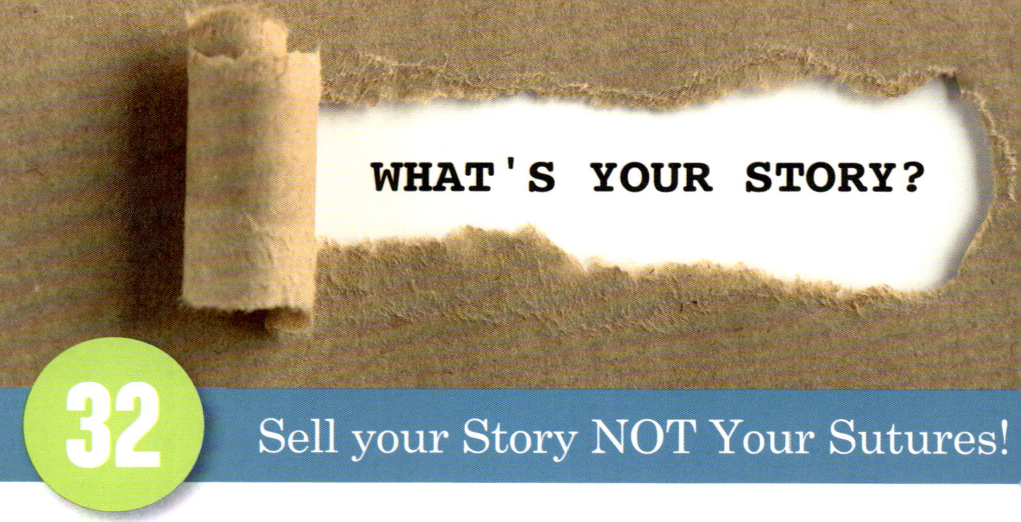

32 Sell your Story NOT Your Sutures!

It's one of the most common marketing mistakes businesses make. The overly aggressive focus on product over brand.

Before you can sell a product effectively, it helps to sell your brand first. What's the story that best speaks to your strengths, your ambition, your goals, etc., etc.? Who do you want to be?

Brands like Apple and Disney come to mind the fastest. Apple built its computer empire by selling an idea along with its products. By personalizing the personal computer, Apple gained an enormous fan base. Likewise Walt Disney shared a similar attention to detail for his amusement parks that Steve Jobs did for Apple's products.

In both cases the brand became synonymous with the men behind the vision. Combined with a solid corporate mission, to some extent, the products began to sell themselves. The question is, how do you market your dental practice in a similar fashion?

One way is to promote your personalized approach. Another might be furthering the dental implant revolution, stressing the psychological and emotional benefits to your patients. If you're a small practice, emphasize your small town roots. If you're a large urban practice, perhaps market your speed and efficiency – a dental practice capable of keeping up with the demands of a fast-moving city.

Your story is unique to you. Once you've nailed it, then you can start selling the sutures – and whatever else your dental practice has in mind.

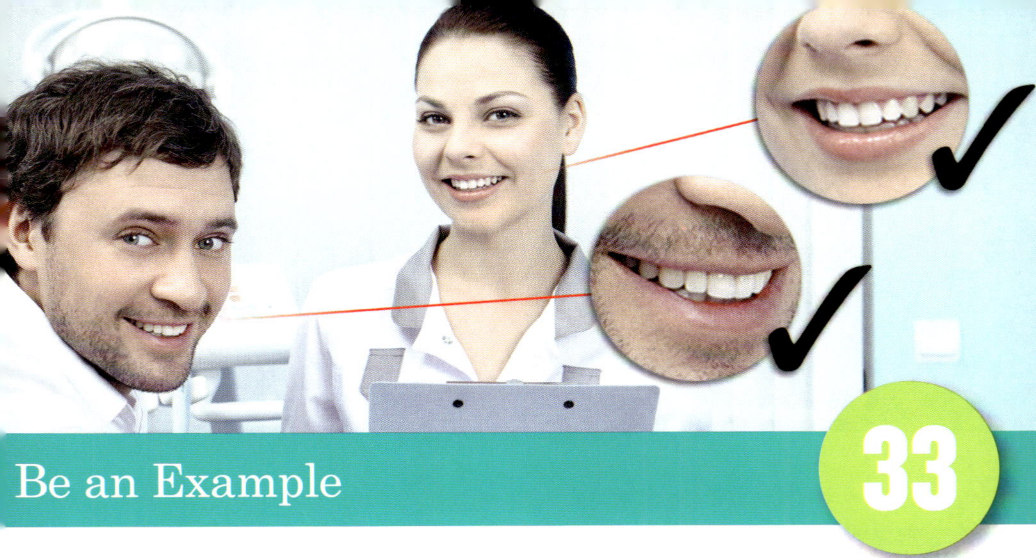

Be an Example

33

A woman and her son made a long train trip to meet with Mahatma Gandhi. After being led to the great leader, she asked him to tell her son that it wasn't healthy to eat candy. Gandhi told her to bring the boy back in two weeks. She reluctantly agreed and made the time-consuming trip back home.

When they returned 14 days later, Gandhi explained to the boy why it was so unhealthy to eat sweets. After the boy left, the mother asked Gandhi why he didn't tell her son that the first time. Gandhi replied, "Because two weeks ago, I was still eating sweets myself."

A year ago I ran into a dentist who was in my graduating class. I was amazed to see the appearance of his teeth. His upper and lower front teeth were severely worn. To add insult to injury, they were crowded and discolored. I didn't say anything, but I was thinking, "And you make recommendations to patients about the health and appearance of their mouths?"

People pay more attention to what you do than what you say. And they pay more attention to who you are than what you do or say. Would you listen to advice given by an overweight family physician or internist who smoked? I doubt it.

On a scale of 1 to 10, rate the health of your mouth and the appearance of your teeth. I hope it's at least a 9. If not, your smile is screaming at your patients, "I don't practice what I preach!" And the same goes for your family and dental team. They're walking billboards for your practice. What do their billboards say? I hope they send messages that influence people to take the actions needed to improve their lives. Because that's the business we dentists are really in.

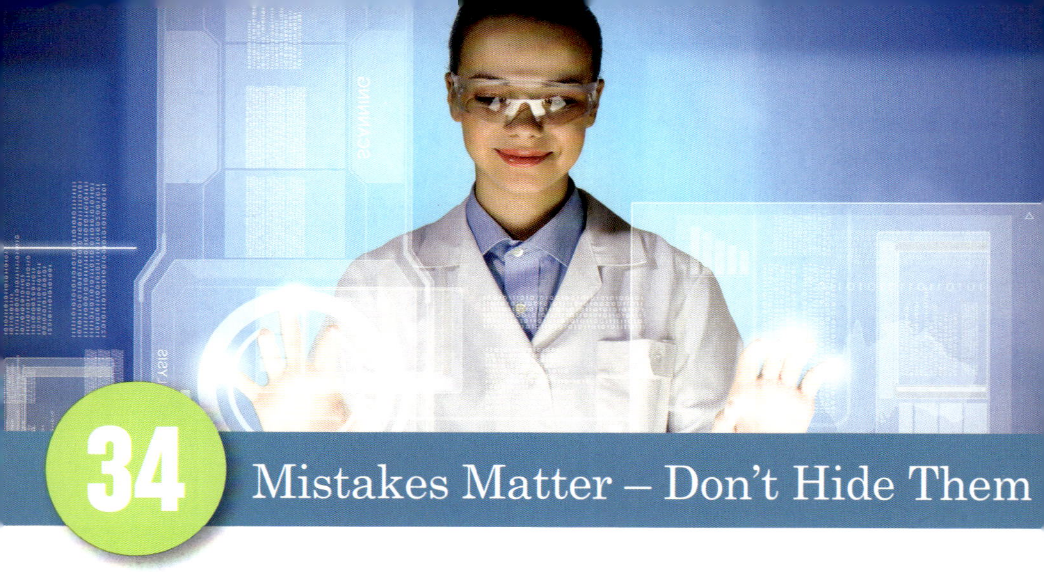

34 Mistakes Matter – Don't Hide Them

Whether you're the boss of your dental practice, a manager at a clothing store, or any other business, mistakes are inevitable.

Admittedly it's not fun when they occur. But the very worst thing you can do is to overreact to them. Chances are the mistake is trivial in comparison to universal issues like life and death. The mistake is also likely small potatoes compared to some of history's greatest corporate blunders.

For instance, did you know that Kodak, the film company, filed a US patent for one of the first digital cameras in 1977? Unfortunately they never released the product to the public. That decision likely cost them billions as the industry converted almost entirely to digital. Or what about the NASA Mars orbiter that was lost in 1999 due to a mismatch between metric and English measurements?

Chances are the blunders your dental staff has made in the past or will make in the future will NOT be this drastic. It helps to keep proper perspective so that when mistakes do happen, you don't overreact.

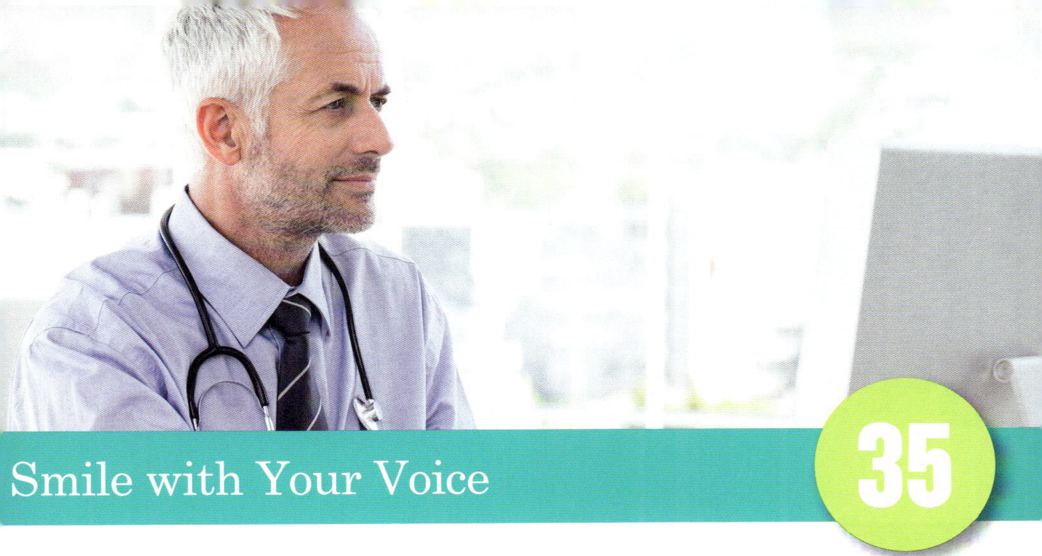

Smile with Your Voice

35

If you read the above title you might be scratching your head. How can one smile with their voice?

Smiling with your voice means being friendly and engaging in person and on the phone. It's more than about just being polite, though. Your warmth, trust, and likability must project through the phone. And in person, the effort can't appear forced. Speak a little slower than you normally would and make sure to articulate your words.

As a social species, we receive a tremendous amount of information through perception. Lacking a complete picture in any given situation we tend to fill in the gaps and make assumptions.

That means that within the first moments of a conversation a patient might wrongly deduce your practice isn't for them – all because a member of the front office staff forgot to smile with their voice.

36 BE AFRAID – Just Don't Be Very Afraid

Unlike the classic Hollywood horror film "The Fly" starring Jeff Goldblum and Geena Davis, being afraid is important – but it's not the be all and end all of the situation at hand.

Being a little afraid is good. Being very afraid is crippling. The key with fear is to channel the emotion into a motivator and not let it prevent forward progress.

Properly channeled, fear can increase alertness, increase reaction time – think the fight or flight response – and it can increase your receptiveness to new ideas and maybe even the need for outside assistance.

How does this apply to the dental office?

Imagine you've just had a less-than-ideal encounter with a patient. Perhaps you even fear the loss of his business. What happens now? If you weren't at least a little fearful of his negative reaction, you wouldn't be motivated to rectify the situation.

Instead, use that fear (maybe this patient will say unkind things about your practice to friends and family) as a vehicle to ensure that whatever has gone wrong in the past with this patient is remedied to the best of your ability.

Throughout human history fear has always had its proper place. And the dental office is as good a place as any to use it to your advantage!

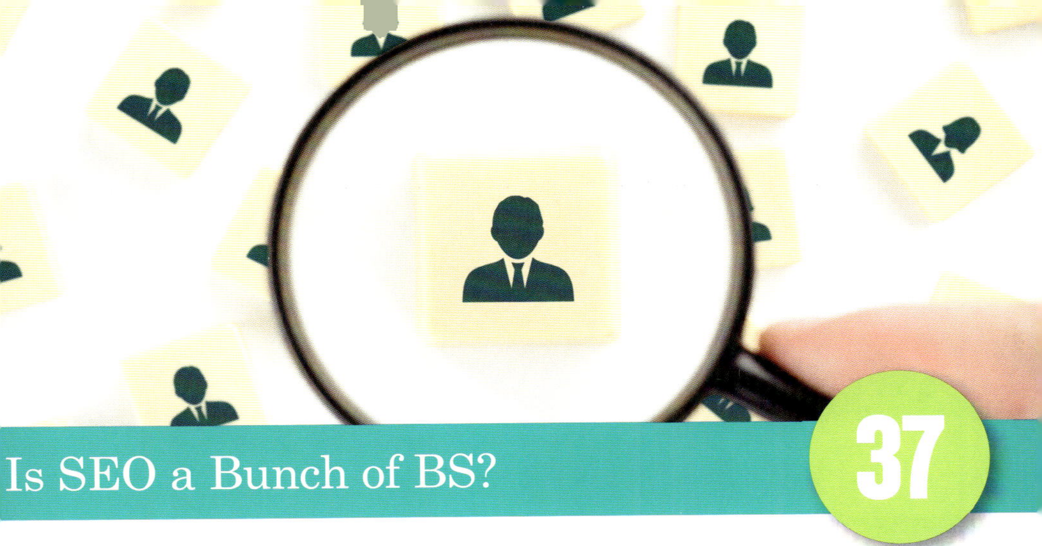

Is SEO a Bunch of BS?

37

To immediately answer the question raised by the title of this tip – no – SEO, or search engine optimization, is not BS. Increasingly it's the way search engine algorithms discover a brand.

Dental practices are no different. They too need to get noticed online. And effective SEO usage – through web content, blogs, articles, etc. – all helps improve your page rankings. Land in the top 10 search hits and you can safely say your business is doing well.

But for all the focus on SEO, don't neglect traditional customer engagement. Create a product that really sells and eventually word of mouth takes over. For dental practices, that could mean the rigorous promotion of a pain-free (or nearly pain-free experience). It could also mean the reliance on cutting-edge imaging technology.

Whatever it is, don't forget to make that your focus and not spin your wheels on excessive SEO.

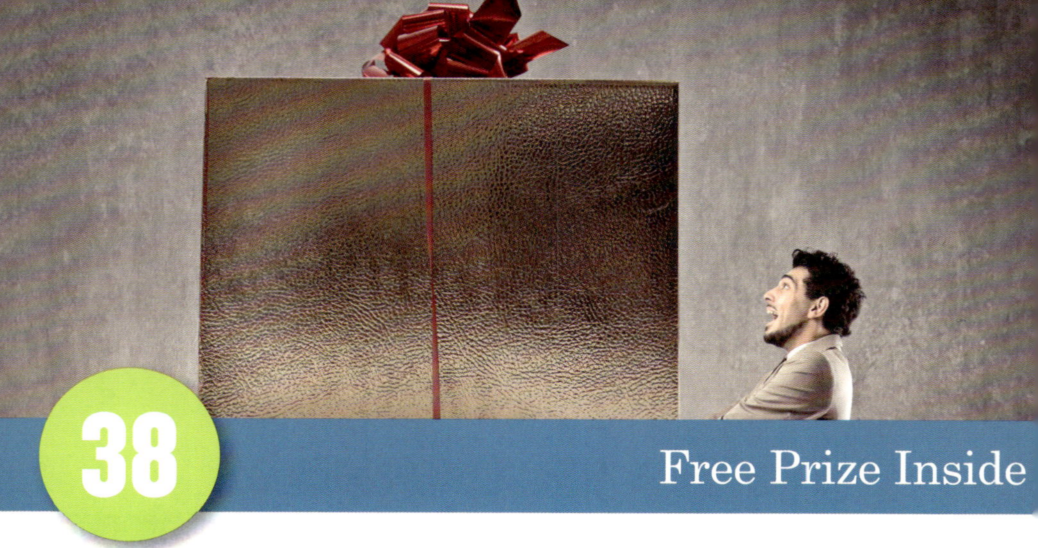

38 Free Prize Inside

When you were a kid, did you buy Cracker Jacks because the product in the box was the best caramel corn; or the least expensive; or the healthiest? Heck no. You bought Cracker Jacks because of the free prize inside the box. The prize was an added benefit that had nothing to do with the product you were buying.

As dentists, our instinct is to believe that the quality of care we provide is the reason patients come to us. This is a distraction from the reality of how people choose when they have choices. We almost never buy the item because the product or service excels at a certain announced metric. Almost no one drives the fastest car. We buy a story. The story is the thing that the product or service also does. It's the other reason we buy something. And usually, the real reason.

Here's an example: You have a seven-year-old daughter. What are you hiring when you select a babysitter? Is it her ability to do CPR, cook gourmet food or teach your little one French? No. You're paying for peace of mind. You're hiring the way it makes you feel to know that someone talented is with your child.

So, great babysitter performance is showing up a few minutes early, dressed appropriately with an air of confidence. Great performance is sending a text every 90 minutes to the concerned parents. Great performance is leaving the kitchen cleaner than it was.

The free prize is the other thing we want to talk about… the prize inside the Cracker Jacks box. That's the story we tell to ourselves and our friends.

What's the free prize in your dental practice's box?

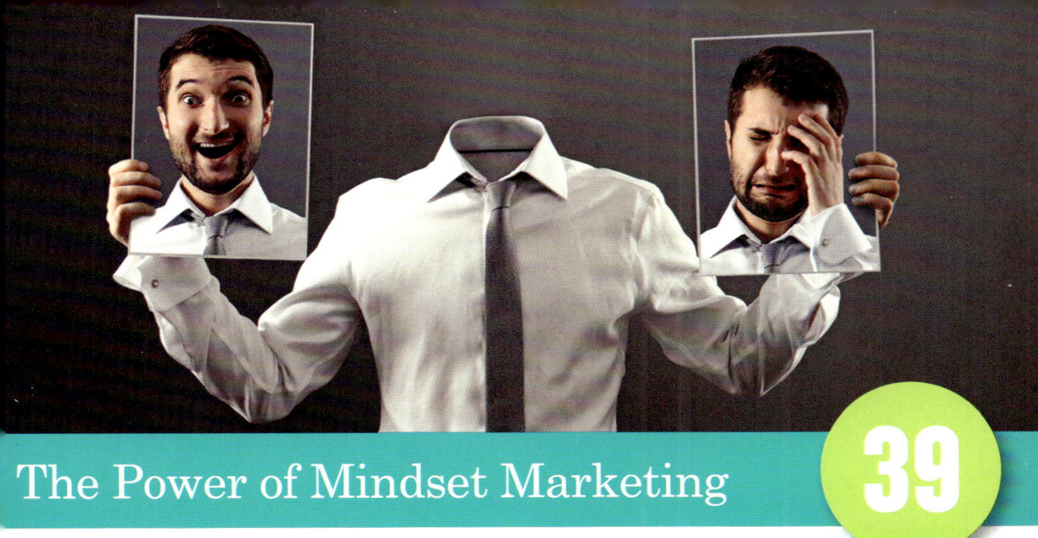

The Power of Mindset Marketing 39

This issue has been raised before, but it bears repeating. In an earlier tip I referenced the importance of storytelling. That in order to sell product en masse, you have to first tell a great story. No argument there.

But there's something subtler that needs to be addressed. What emotions are you trying to sell? What's the power level of your mindset marketing?

Often I analogize this to buying a car. Rare is the customer who truly goes out and purchases the "best" vehicle. Measured in terms of top speed, acceleration, safety and overall performance, these tangible metrics are but one component to why people purchase the car of their choice.

They buy the car because of how it makes them feel. For some that means feeling "cool." For others it means feeling "safe." The trick is to market a vehicle to a potential buyer and help elicit that emotion.

So how does a dental practice elicit an emotional response? Surprisingly, the car comparison still applies. For instance, thanks in part to the burgeoning popularity of cosmetic dentistry and smile design, what's your dental practice cool factor?

It may sound odd to talk about a dental office's coolness, but it really is the case. Sell that appeal. Market it. Promote in online. Talk up your practice with your friends and colleagues, maybe even buy that new car you were talking about. Especially in an urban area, which tends to congregate more fashion-conscious people, having a great smile is as important as having a great body.

But the suburbs and rural areas shouldn't feel left out. Mindset marketing knows no limits. Perhaps for your dental practice, peace of mind is your top selling point. Maybe you've been in practice for decades and watched young patients mature, get married, have children of their own, and still they're patients at your practice.

Whatever your mindset is, make sure to telegraph that idea as part of your overall story. Remember, a great story sells, but all great stories germinate from great ideas!

Think about that the next time you talk about your practice, your passion, and how with each patient you treat, little by little, you're transforming a life!

Pretty cool, huh?!?!

40 Think Beyond Brick-and-Mort

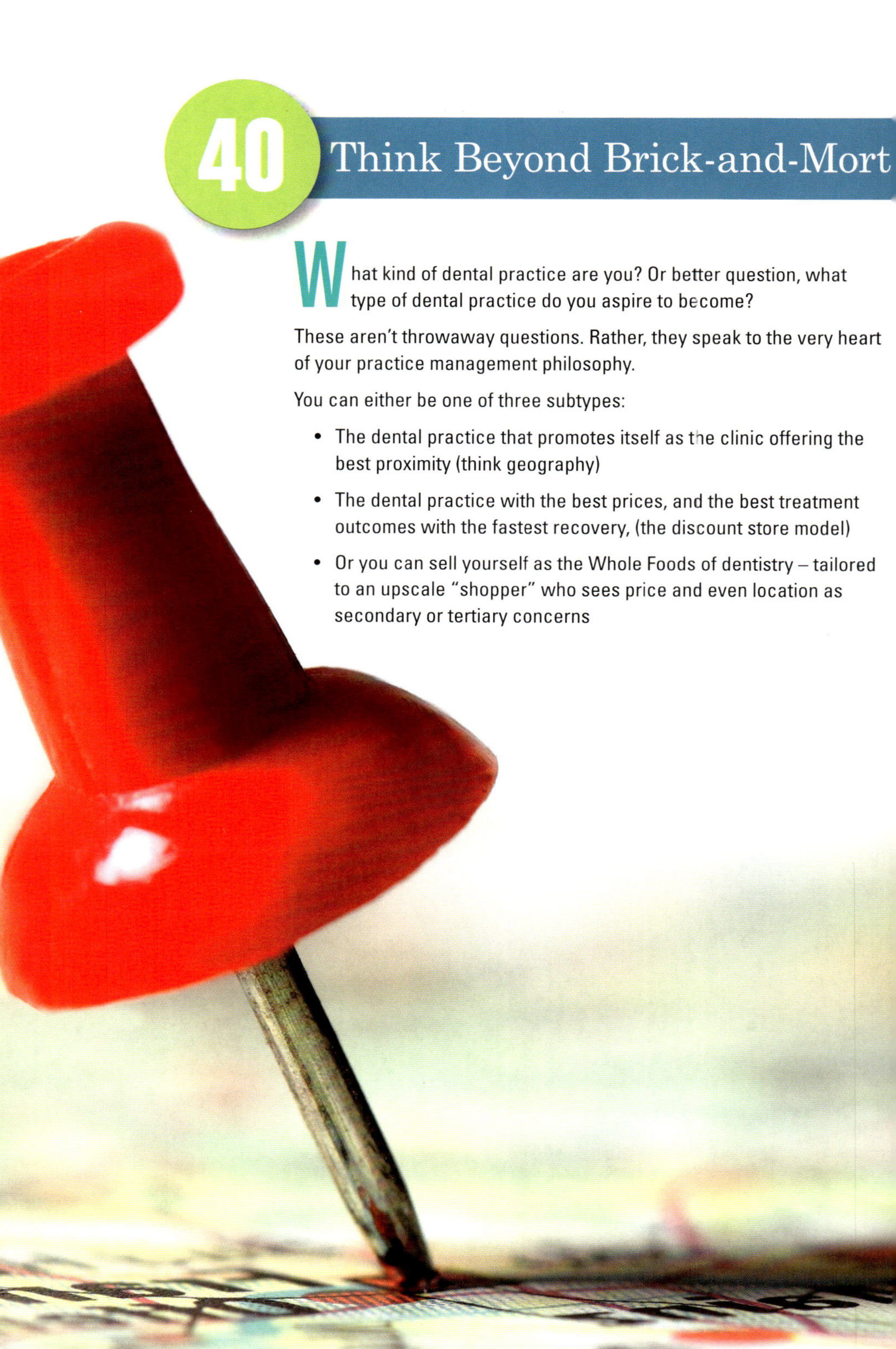

What kind of dental practice are you? Or better question, what type of dental practice do you aspire to become?

These aren't throwaway questions. Rather, they speak to the very heart of your practice management philosophy.

You can either be one of three subtypes:

- The dental practice that promotes itself as the clinic offering the best proximity (think geography)
- The dental practice with the best prices, and the best treatment outcomes with the fastest recovery, (the discount store model)
- Or you can sell yourself as the Whole Foods of dentistry – tailored to an upscale "shopper" who sees price and even location as secondary or tertiary concerns

It's virtually impossible for a single dental practice to fit all three categories. When they do, it's likely they're trying too hard, and again falling into the trap of being too many things for too many people.

If you're a larger operation with several clinics perhaps you can tweak your practices in such a way as to hit the mark in multiple areas. That's true especially if your clinics are separated by more than a few miles and cross significant socio-economic segments of your community.

Otherwise, employ the KISS philosophy (not the band) and Keep It Simple, Stupid. Pursue one model at a time and take the time needed to evaluate and measure its success. Like any business, key performance indicators (KPIs) should be tracked on a weekly, monthly, quarterly and yearly basis.

If, however, after a given interval you see that the current model isn't attracting, retaining and engaging new patients, consider an alternative. This is also what it means to think beyond brick-and-mortar. While your typical patient won't travel more than, say, 15-20 miles to your dental office, here is where the web is a vital tool. Your online marketing can and should be a vital tool in promoting the type of dental practice you envision yourself becoming. Doing so will help push the boundaries of the above-referenced travel radius. It's also a great place to offer promotions and other price incentives to certain kinds of patients – especially if you're aiming for "discount dentistry."

Whichever course you choose don't be afraid to fail! Think beyond traditional brick-and-mortar and your patients – new ones and old ones alike – will thank you that you did!

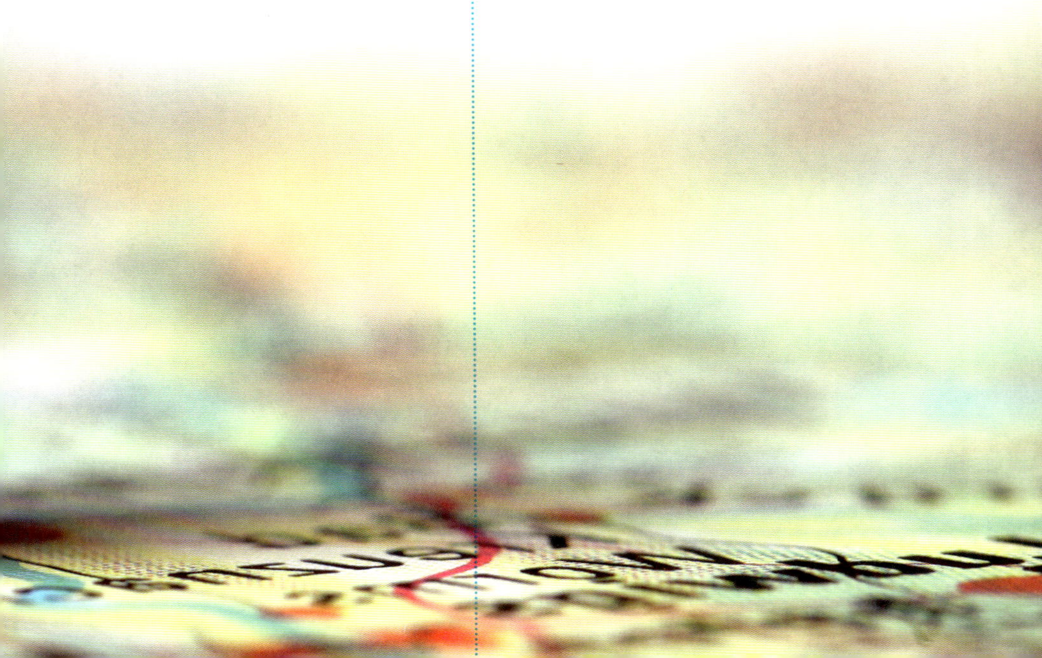

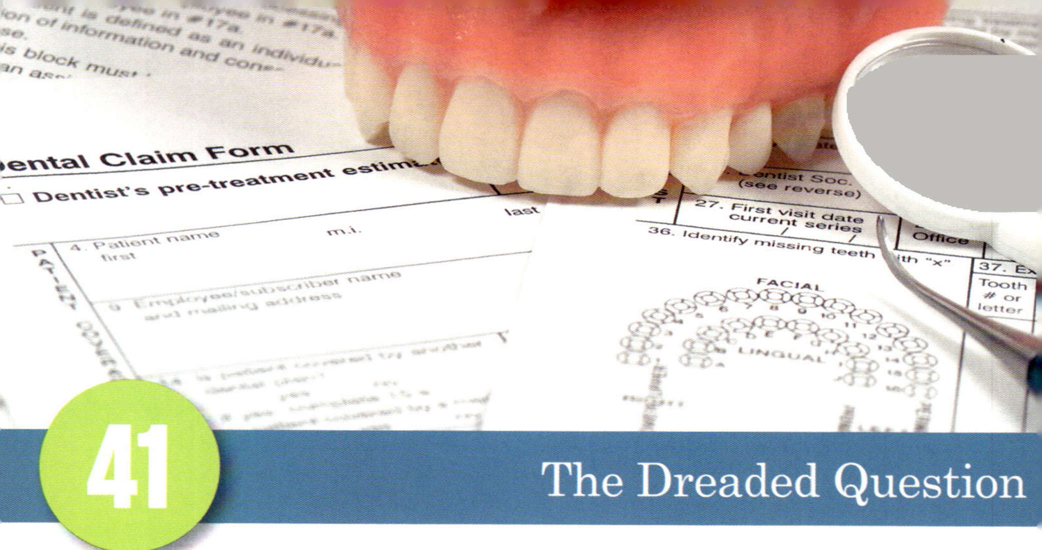

41 The Dreaded Question

It is a dark and stormy morning. The clouds are building on the horizon. Lightning begins to light up the sky. The air is still and silent. It is a day only Freddie Kruger could love.

Your office phone rings. The entire team stares at it with dread in their eyes. Finally, your front desk person musters the nerve to pick it up. Everyone holds their breath. Through the speaker phone, The Dreaded Question pierces your ear drum. "Do you take my insurance? It's called The Most Horrible HMO Ever."

If you don't accept this stellar plan, how do you answer the caller's question? Most people simply say, "No," and the conversation screeches to an abrupt halt. Now, they won't have access to your outstanding care, and you lose a patient.

Here's another way to answer the "Do you take my insurance? It's called The Most Horrible HMO Ever" question. Just reply, "Mrs. Jones, that's an excellent question. Thanks for asking. We aren't a member of your plan, but we do see many patients with that insurance. We will work with you to maximize your benefits. That way you can still receive the high quality care we offer." Now explain how the process works in your practice.

Your goal is to be completely honest and inform patients that they can still come to your office. And always stress the great care they will receive from you.

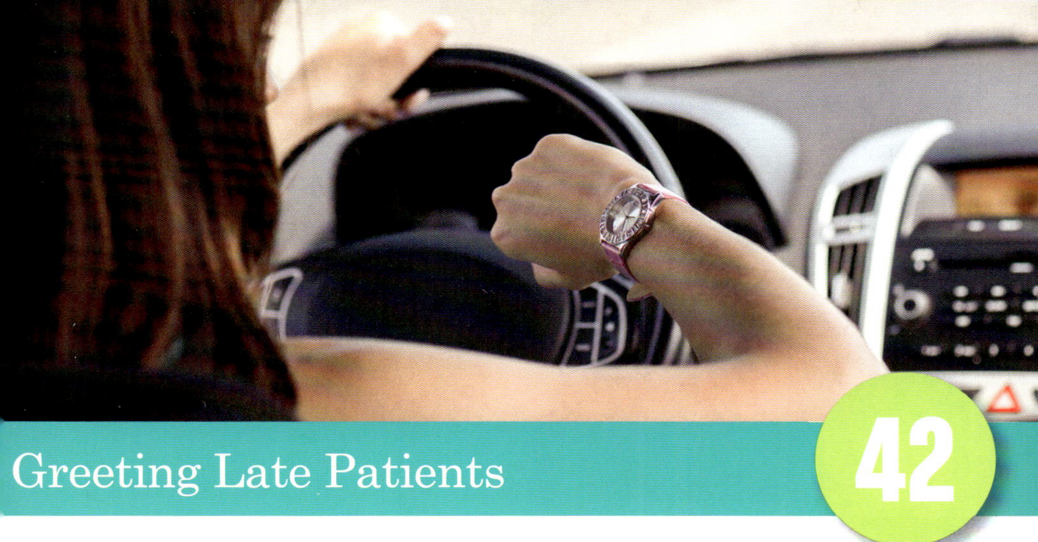

Greeting Late Patients

42

You need to handle late patients with courtesy and at the same time maintain control of your schedule. Here is a great way to do it:

Patient: "Sorry I'm late."

Team Member: "I hope everything is okay. We were worried about you."

Patient: "The traffic was horrible."

Team Member: "I understand. As you know, we pride ourselves on running on time. We scheduled 60 minutes for your visit, and we need every minute of that time to complete your restoration. We want to make sure you receive the very best care we can offer. Let me check to see that there is still enough time available."

Four additional distinctions:

1. It's very important to stay on schedule the majority of the time. If you're always running late, you will train your patients to be late too.
2. Another way to train tardiness is to say, "That's okay. We'll get you right in" after a patient arrives late.
3. If a patient is five minutes late, call them and say, "Hi Mary, this is Doris from Dr. Garg's office. We were expecting to see you at 10. We're concerned that something happened. Please call us right away."
4. If there isn't enough time to do the entire planned procedure for the late patient, maybe you can complete a portion of the care.

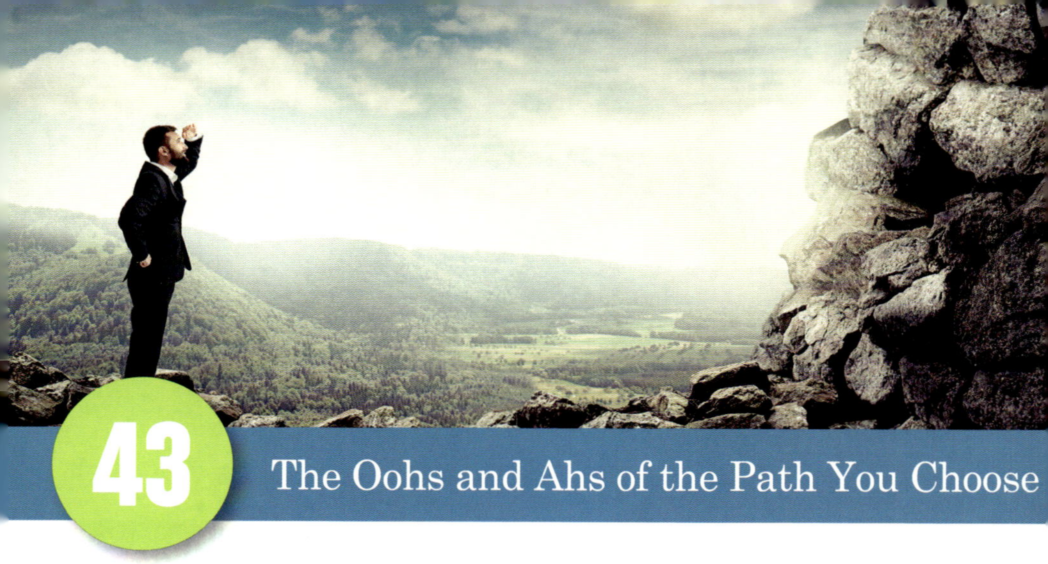

43 The Oohs and Ahs of the Path You Choose

All paths in life have what I call "ooh" and "ah" moments. Moments that annoy – the oohs – and moments that excite – the ahs.

Choosing the right path for you comes down to a cost-benefit analysis. The closer we get toward the path of least resistance but with the highest rewards, the happier we'll be.

But in life it's also true that paths with the greatest risk often net the greatest reward.

The path you choose is entirely up to you. Dentistry certainly has plenty of ah moments. Just remember that it's natural to experience bumps along the road.

Let them be teachable moments and not cause for a detour.

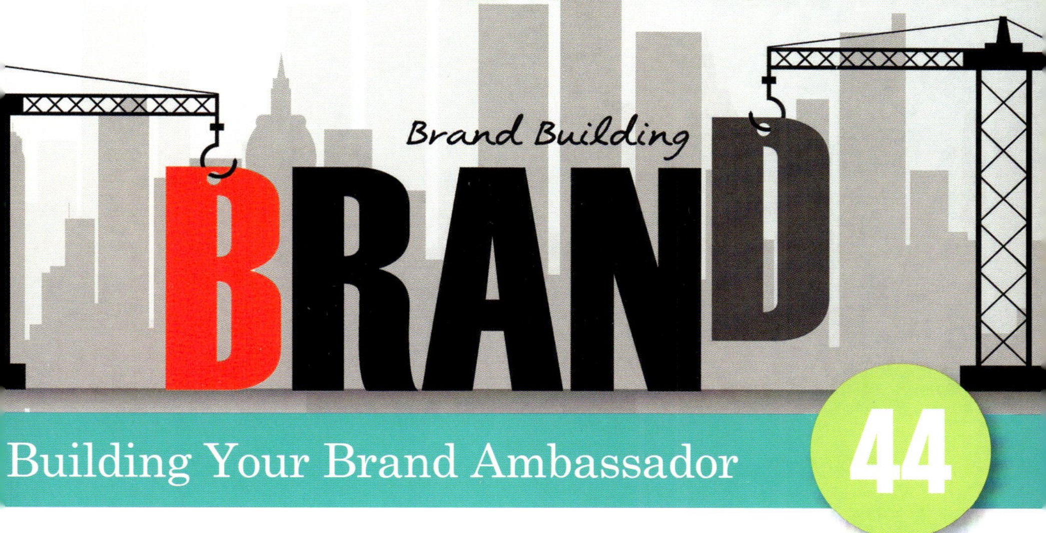

44 Building Your Brand Ambassador

Brand ambassador is a term you might have heard before. Rarely, though, has it been applied to dentistry.

That is, until now!

Brand ambassadors are your most loyal customers. These are the men and women, who, thanks to a combination of reasons, are eager to support your cause – sometimes for very little in return – at least in the immediate.

Thanks to years of superior customer service and customer engagement, these people will go through the proverbial fire with you. As loyal customers, they're unlikely to leave your brand even if indisputable facts suggest there's a better deal, a better offer, or a better product right around the corner.

These are special people. And all brands should be proud of themselves for having cultivated such a dedicated group.

Dental practices should strive to think similarly. Cultivate your own "rock stars" and use their endorsement as a vehicle to attract new patients. One of the best ways to do this is of course by word of mouth. Even a friendly reminder from someone on your staff to one of these individuals encouraging a conversation could be a huge success.

I'm also a big fan of testimonials – either written and published on your website, or recorded in video format. Consider upping the experience further by having a videographer (freelance or in-house, depending on your needs and the size of your business) conduct a question-and-answer style interview. Done right, it could bring a degree of professionalism to the endorsement.

Regardless of which approach you take, remember that dental practices at the end of the day, operate like any business. And your brand ambassadors can help you transform your practice.

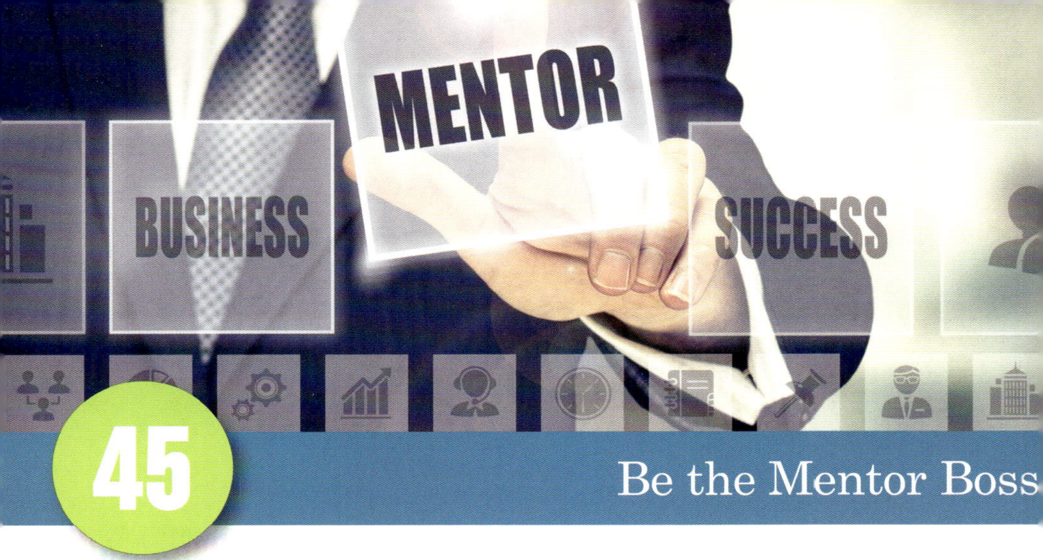

45 Be the Mentor Boss

There's an expression to which all business leaders can relate: "it's lonely at the top."

Bosses, by the very definition of the term, are a select group of people who oversee others. Very often the position lends itself to isolation. Some things just can't be shared with subordinates, no matter how close the relationship can seem.

Good bosses are good leaders – men and women who lead by example, are flexible and forgiving when they need to be, matter-of-fact and critical when they have to be.

But can bosses be more than that?

Yes they can!

How?

By taking on mentor-like attributes. The dictionary defines a mentor as "a wise and trusted counselor or teacher."

Ideally you want your dental staff not only to respect you, but learn from you as well. And better still, be inspired by you. If your staff already sees you in a mentor-like light, chances are you'll be able to execute better leadership. Employees who feel like they're being mentored will also be more receptive to criticism because they know and trust the feedback is coming from a good place.

Bear this in mind as you mold your dental practice in your image. It might always be lonely at the top. But if you're loved by your staff, chances are that loneliness will be a little less acute.

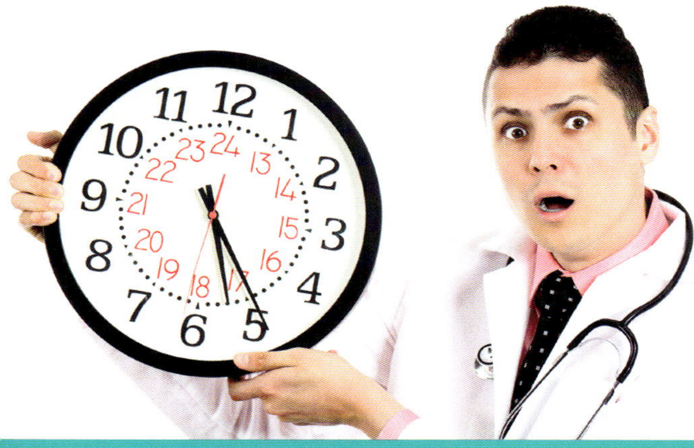

Late in the Day Emergency Conversation 46

It's 4:59 pm. You're just about to walk out the door on Friday after a full day in the office. The phone rings. You think, "Should I pick it up or not?" Being a dedicated professional, you snatch the phone off its cradle at the last possible second. And you hear this: "I have a tooth that's killing me! I need to see a dentist immediately!"

One of your options would be to say, "You have the wrong number. No dentists live here." Another option is to have the following conversation:

Team member: "Let me see how I can help you. When was your last visit with us?" If they are a patient of record, you may want to see them that day. If not and they say:

Patient: "I haven't been to your office before."

Team Member: "I'm sorry to hear about your tooth. I wish you would have called us earlier so we could have helped you. We gladly see emergencies every day during regular office hours. Unfortunately, our office is closing now and the doctor won't be available until Monday."

Patient: "So what should I do?"

Team Member: "We would be happy to see you on Monday. Or you can call dental office ABC that has evening hours. Their number is 555-5555. Which would you prefer?"

Four additional distinctions:

1. Your team members must know how you want these types of calls to be handled. And they need to have a script memorized.
2. If you do wish to see these end-of-the-day emergencies, the team needs to know how to schedule them and what additional "after-hours" fee is required. Seeing emergencies is an excellent way to build your practice.
3. If patients are seen after hours, payment in full should be arranged over the phone. Insurance should be submitted for the patient to be reimbursed directly.
4. If patients call you at home, and they are not patients of record, simply say, "I'm sorry that I can't see you today." Then ask them to call your office in the morning or refer them to someone who may be able to help them immediately.

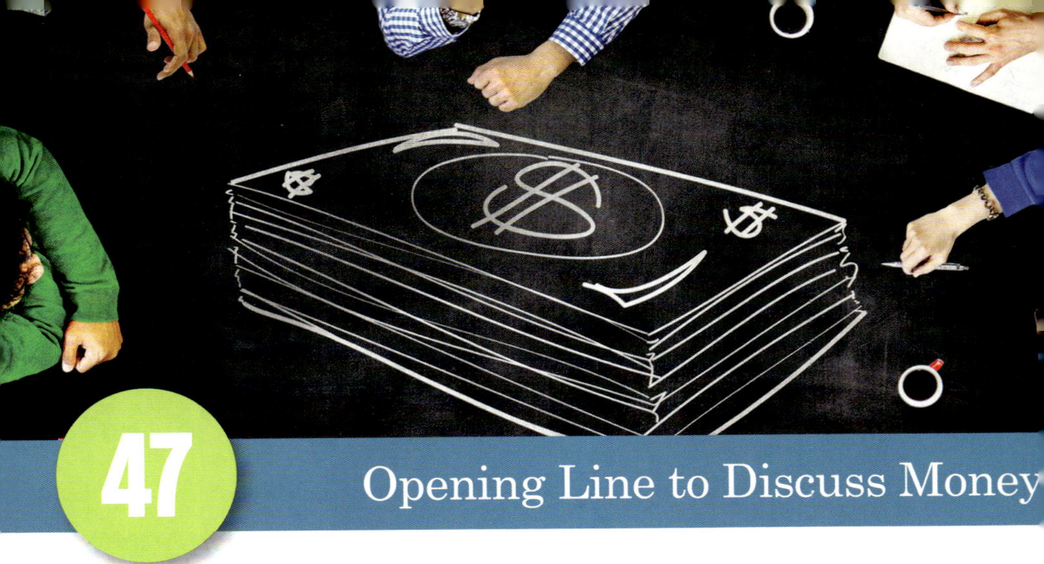

47 Opening Line to Discuss Money

For most dental team members, discussing money with patients is a difficult conversation. As a result, they tend to put off these conversations or begin them awkwardly.

As described in my book, Implant Excellence, money should be discussed as early as possible so your patients are not shocked with the fees you quote. If you have done your job effectively, the patient's reaction to your treatment plan fees should be, "That's about what I thought it would be."

An excellent way to begin to talk about money early is to ask your new patients this question: "Is there anything that would stand in your way of getting the dental care you need and desire?" Of course, have these kinds of conversations in a private setting. If they mention that finances could be a challenge for them, discuss the different payment options you have. As an example:

- A 5% accounting reduction for payment made before treatment is started.
- Visa, MasterCard or Amex
- No interest options for up to 24 months
- Payment plans with interest for up to 60 months

With your new or old patients, after a fee has been quoted, use this line as an opening to discuss money: "José, I'd like to help you with the fee for your treatment and talk with you about the payment options we have. Let's see what will work best for you. OK?"

Almost everyone will say, "Yes." This small "yes" is more important than you might imagine. When answering in the affirmative, they make a small step toward case acceptance. And a series of small steps toward making a big purchase is way better than one big leap – which is how most dental offices do it.

A few people will say, "No." This will signal you to step back and discuss what is holding them back from making a decision. It's much better to have this conversation now than to have it after you've spent time and effort explaining fees and payment options.

Be confident. Be brave. Be successful. Don't be afraid to discuss money. Bring it up before you have to. Everyone will benefit.

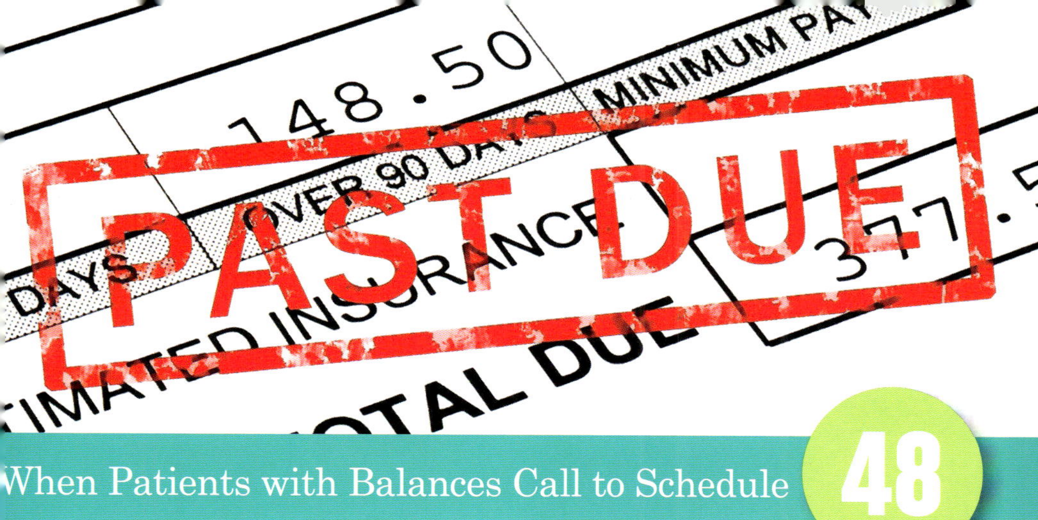

When Patients with Balances Call to Schedule 48

When patients call to schedule, and they have a balance on their accounts, you want to accomplish two objectives:

1. Collect your money
2. Keep them as patients (perhaps with some new payment guidelines)

With these objectives in mind, here's how the call should go:

Patient: "I had a molar pulled last year in your office. And I need another one pulled now. It's killing me."

Team Member: "I'd be happy to help you with that. Dr. Lopez can see you this afternoon. I see that our records show you have a balance on your account. Let me help you with a way to clear up this balance and take care of the fee for today's visit."

Patient: "I thought I paid last time."

Team Member: "Our records show a balance of $80 on your account. We ask that you clear up this balance and take care of today's fees before your visit this afternoon. We accept Visa, MasterCard, Amex, check or cash. Which will work best for you?"

Three Additional Distinctions:

1. When patients of record call to schedule visits, check their records to make sure their balances are paid.
2. Explain why there is a balance if they ask. Most people won't ask.
3. If patients have shown they are not timely with their payments, be certain they pay BEFORE any care is provided.

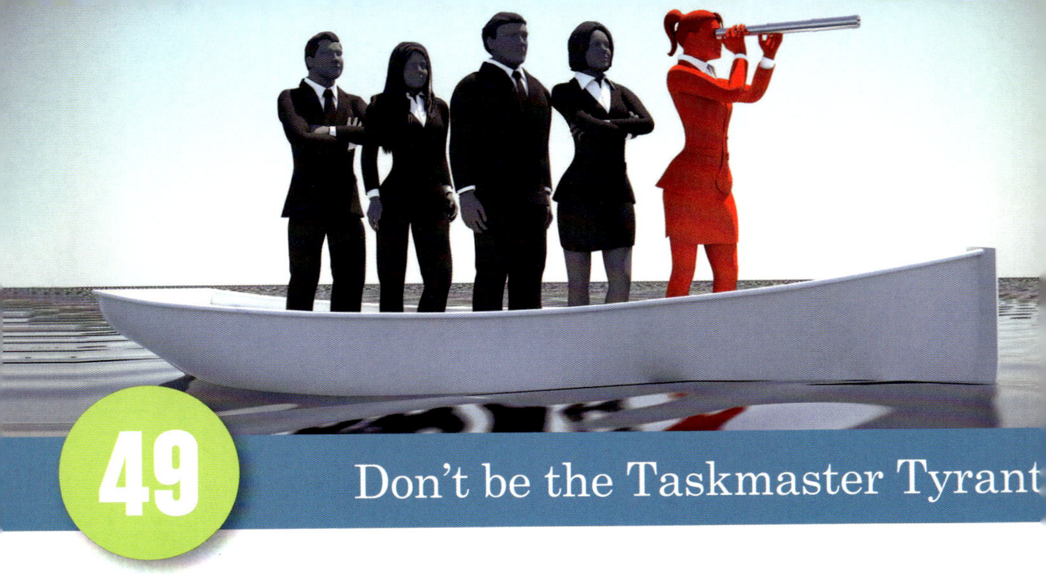

49 Don't be the Taskmaster Tyrant

If tip 45 encouraged you to be the "mentor boss" it's natural, then, to have a tip about what kind of boss you shouldn't be – especially when it comes to running a successful dental practice.

Above all, don't become what I call a "taskmaster tyrant." In today's services-based and information age economy, taskmaster tyrants limit creative thinking, they suffocate out-of-the-box ideas, and they generally create loyalty through fear rather than inspiration. That means low office morale. And it's a condition your patients will easily recognize.

Don't get me wrong, historically these kinds of bosses had their time and place. Industrial jobs still require a steady hand. So too do positions that require exceptional organization and with a company with lots of moving parts.

A dental practice, even a larger one, is more simplistic. Don't treat your team members like standardized car parts, treat them as individuals. Don't constantly throw it back in their faces that you pay their salaries and therefore they are subject to your every whim. Don't micromanage. And don't micromanage with the fear that even the slightest mistake will result in termination.

Walking the line between disciplinarian and inspirational leader can be difficult. But if you have to choose one side to err on, I'd choose inspirational leader any day!

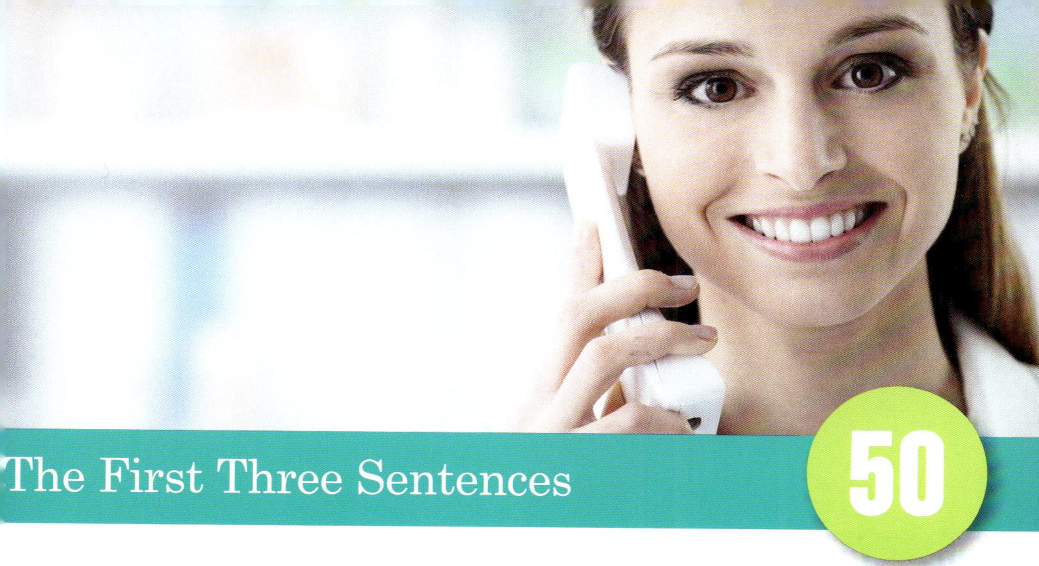

50 The First Three Sentences

The first three sentences your patients hear when calling your office are vitally important. They set the tone for the rest of the conversation. When well constructed, these three sentences will:

- positively differentiate you from other offices
- enhance your level of rapport and trust
- reinforce their decision for calling you

The first three sentences I suggest using are: "Thank you for calling Dr. Garg's office. This is Darlene. I can help you."

Sentence #1 - "Thank you for calling Dr. Garg's office."

Always use the same opening line so you don't stumble around with the likes of, "Good morning…er… ah… I mean good afternoon." It's always appropriate to thank people because your kids don't eat if the patients don't come in.

Sentence #2 - "This is Darlene."

When the team member answering the phone identifies herself, it personalizes the conversation and helps the caller be more comfortable.

Sentence #3 - "I can help you."

The statement "I can help you" establishes a more positive tone to the call than the question "How can I help you?" And your practice can always help callers even if it's answering a question or referring them to some other office.

At your next team meeting, emphasize why phone skills are so important and have everyone role play the First Three Sentences at least 10 times.

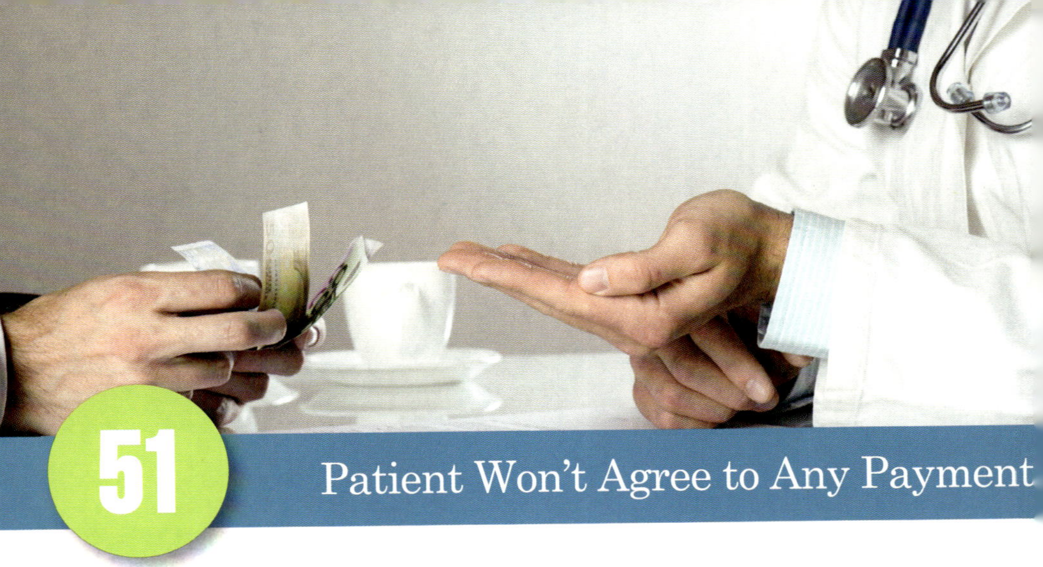

51 Patient Won't Agree to Any Payment

You will usually receive an answer when you ask patients, "Which of the four payment options works best for you?" But occasionally, you will hear:

Patient: "None of these options work for me. What should I do?"

Team Member: "I understand and really want to help you. Let me be sure I covered every option we have available." Now, the team member describes the options again using different words.

Patient: "I don't think I can do any of them."

Team Member: "I appreciate how hard it can be to find a way to make this work. I'm happy to continue to explore options that have worked for other patients who had similar concerns."

Patient: "Guess I need to think about it."

Team Member: "It's your decision. I'm always here to help you whatever you decide. Please call me if your circumstances change, and you want to explore possibilities. For now, let's get you scheduled for your recare visit."

Patient: "OK."

Team Member: "And is it OK if I follow-up with you in a week or so to see if circumstances have changed?"

Patient: "Sure."

Four Additional Distinctions:

1. Always stay on the patient's side. Never make it an "us versus you" conversation.
2. In different words, review your payment options a second time.
3. Respectfully acknowledge the patient's decision, and assure them that you are always available to talk.
4. Emphasize that this is not the end of your relationship. Make sure you get them back for a recare visit.

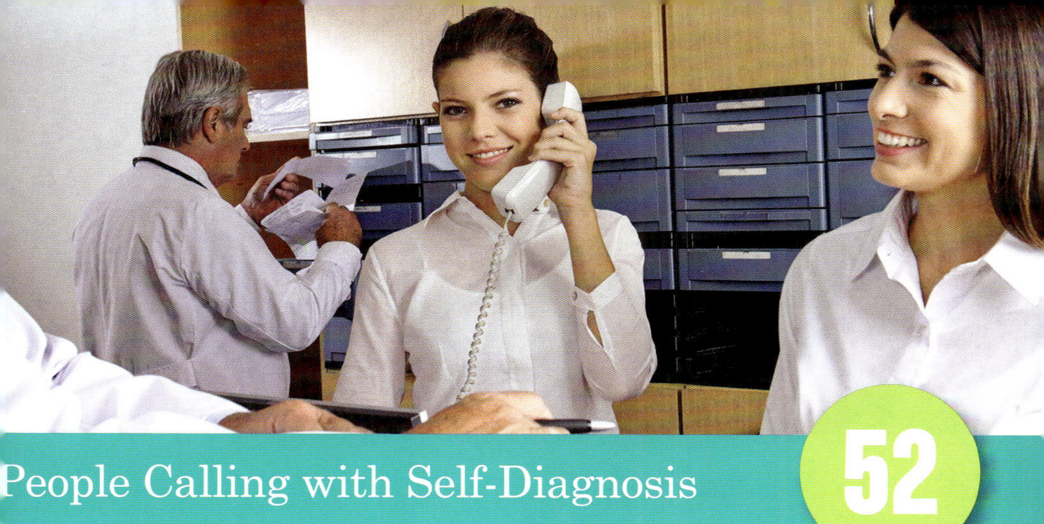

People Calling with Self-Diagnosis 52

People may call your office with their own treatment diagnosis. Your goals should be to help the caller and maintain productive schedule. To accomplish this, olitely communicate that a proper diagnosis s needed. This will avoid scheduling reatment time that might not be needed.

ere is one way the conversation should roceed:

aller: "I broke my tooth and need a filling."

eam Member: "I can help you with that. Do ou have any discomfort?"

aller: "No. Just need the tooth filled."

eam Member: "The doctor can see you this norning at 11 or tomorrow at 3. Which time is est for you?"

aller: "Tomorrow at 3."

Team Member: "Excellent. Here's how the doctor will help you. We'll take an x-ray of the area and the doctor will examine the tooth. Once Dr. Johnson has made a diagnosis, she will recommend the care you need."

Caller: "I don't need all that other stuff. I just want my tooth filled."

Team Member: "I understand. A broken tooth sometimes needs more than a filling. The doctor will need to see the x-ray and check the tooth to determine what treatment is best for you."

Caller: "OK."

When you handle the call this way, you don't offend the caller AND you make sure your procedures are followed. Everybody wins.

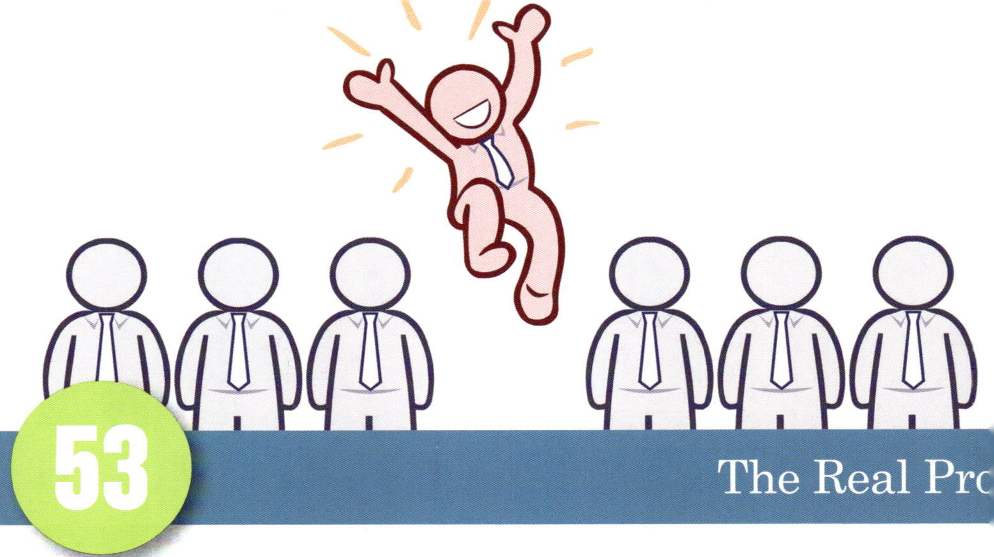

53 The Real Pro

Every profession creates them. The Real Pro is on one side of the chasm and the Average Joe is on the other. The Real Pro knows how to walk, talk and engage with people in ways that amplify their professionalism.

Average Joe dentists aren't necessarily that way because they aren't talented. It's merely because they haven't invested the time or found the motivation to cross the chasm to the side of the Real Pros.

It's fun to make a fish-out-of-water movie about outsiders who are excellent at their craft. But in real life, fish out of water don't do very well. To be financially successful in dentistry, being a Real Pro might be even more important than actually being good at what you do. I firmly believe you should do both. Have the skills, the team and the practice that delivers excellent quality dentistry to your patients AND present yourself as a Real Pro.

The people in your community can easily spo the Real Pro dentists, are more apt to visit their office and accept the care presented. On which side of the chasm will you decide to stand?

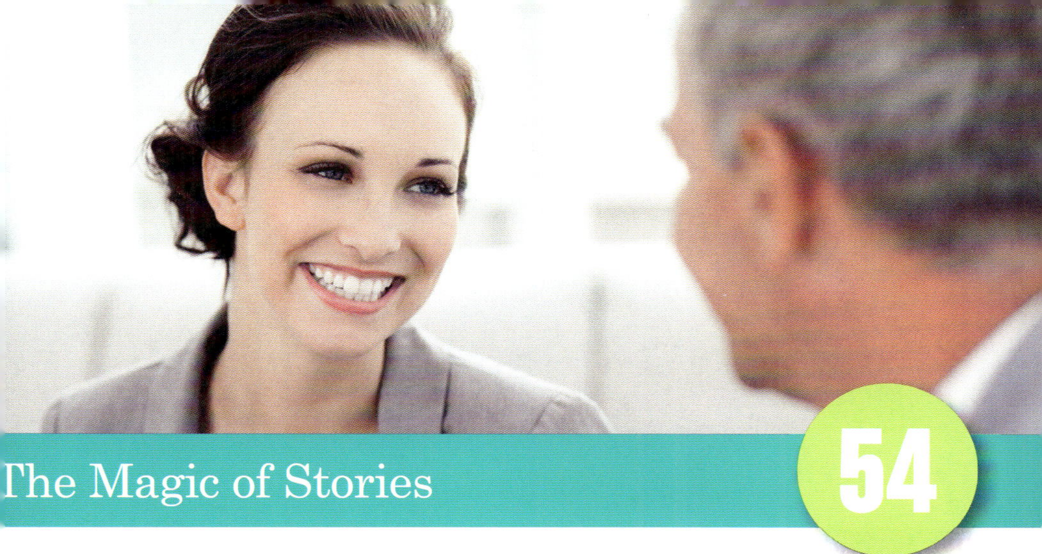

The Magic of Stories 54

eadership maven, Tom Peters, said, "The best leaders . . . almost without exception and at every level, are master users of tories and symbols." Tom is right. Stories re magic. They are the natural medium to onvey messages of any type to any person r group... your family, dental team and atients.

ll effective stories have three parts – eginning, middle and end. In the beginning f the story, we learn about the central haracter's normal world, what her elationships are like and what challenges he faces.

the middle of a story, the central character ttempts to solve the challenges. Sometimes he succeeds. Sometimes she doesn't. But he learns valuable lessons on her journey.

the end of a story, the central character athers all she has learned and takes ffective and decisive action to succeed... which she does in almost all stories.

When you want to communicate a course of action for patients in your dental practice, tell a story about a patient who was in a similar situation (beginning); the action they took (middle) and the positive result they achieved (ending). The patients will get into the story. They will identify with the central character, vicariously learn the vital lessons and be more apt to take the same actions.

When you communicate with others, ask yourself three questions:

1. Did they understand what you said?
2. Did they believe it?
3. Will they remember it?

Stories will do all three. So, create a collection of powerful stories. Then tell each story at just the right time. Those around you will be moved to improve and your life will be enhanced.

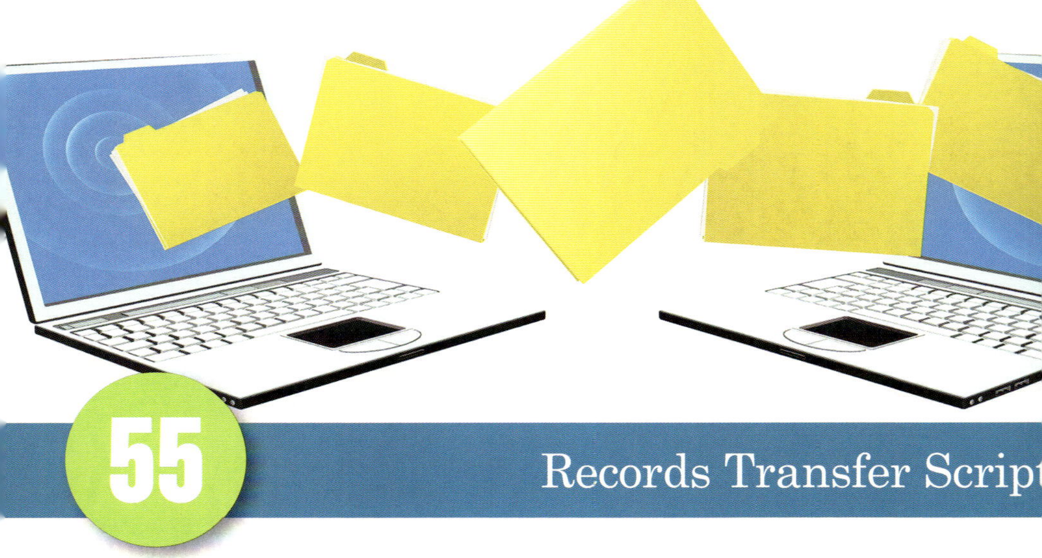

55 Records Transfer Script

When a patient requests a transfer of their records, use the following script:

Patient: "I would like my records transferred to another dental office."

Team Member: "I can help you with that. What is the name and address of the office?"

Patient: "Send them to Dr. Pam Skillet at 111 Main Street."

Team Member: "How soon will you be seeing Dr. Skillet?"

Patient: "Next January."

Team Member: "We will miss you. May I ask why you're leaving?"

Patient: "We're moving and her office is a lot closer to our new home."

Team Member: "I understand. I wanted to be sure you were happy with the care and service we've given you. You're always welcome to return."

Comments:

1. Don't assume the reason for leaving is because they are dissatisfied with you.
2. Quickly collect the transfer information.
3. If they are dissatisfied with you, discover the reason and make amends if needed.
4. Express that you are sorry to see them go.
5. Convey that they are welcome back at any time.

Always provide excellent service to people even when they are leaving the practice. It's the right thing to do, and they may be back some day… or refer others to you.

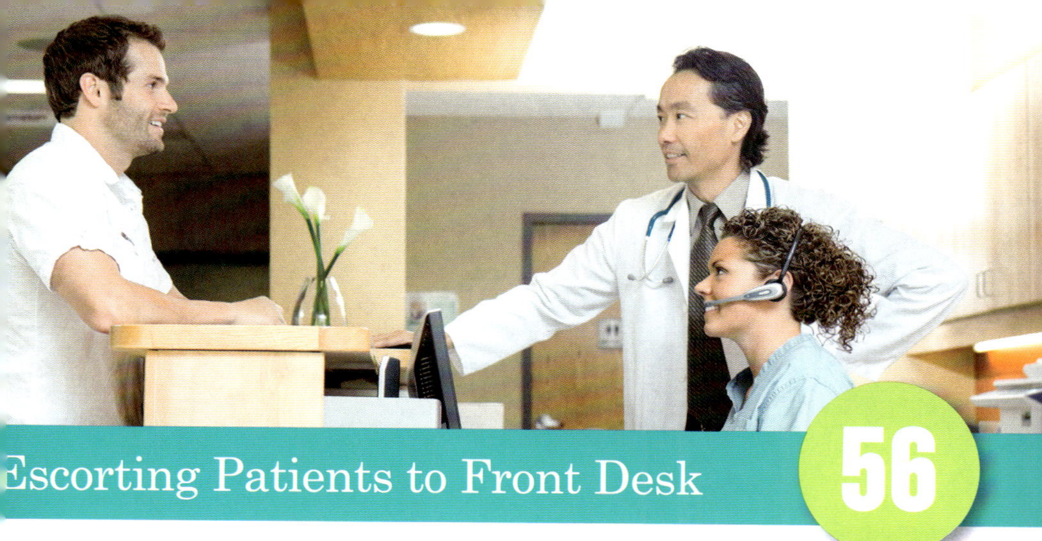

Escorting Patients to Front Desk 56

One often overlooked time to have a valuable conversation is when your treatment assistants, hygienists or you escort patients to the front desk. Here is an effective sample conversation:

Team Member: "Mark, I will escort you to the front desk to see Monique. She will schedule your next visit and review the fee for your treatment and our payment options."

When the team member and patient reach the front desk, the team member makes an effective hand-off.

Team Member: "Monique, Mark has agreed to have two, very large, broken-down metal fillings replaced with porcelain crowns. He is aware that the investment is $2,200. Please explain to Mark our payment options and schedule his two visits as soon as possible. Mark, we'll see you again in a couple of weeks."

Three Additional Distinctions:

1. Don't allow patients to wander by themselves to the front desk. Escort them so the front desk person can properly complete their visit.
2. It's much easier for your front desk person to discuss fees if patients know the conversation is about to occur.
3. Smart dental practices use every opportunity to have meaningful conversations with patients. The short trip to the front desk can be one of them.

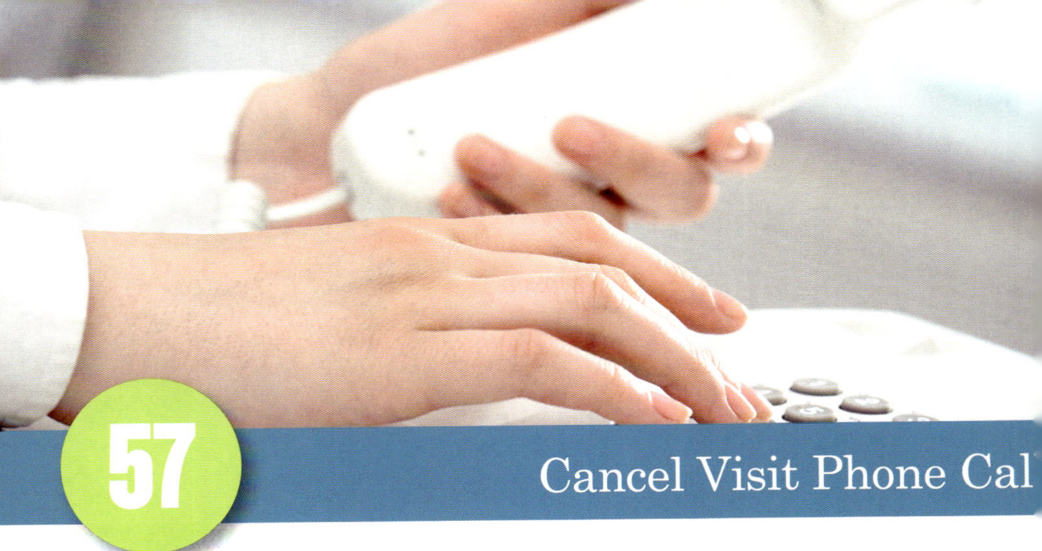

57 Cancel Visit Phone Cal

Cancellation phone calls from your patients must be handled well because you are trying to accomplish two outcomes at one time:

1. Get the patients rescheduled
2. Let them know that most late cancellations are not good for them or you

Here's how an effective conversation should go followed by important points to consider:

Patient: "I need to cancel my appointment this afternoon. I had an emergency come up."

Team Member: "I'm sorry to hear that. We have a waiting list of people who really want to get in, but with such short notice, we won't be able to contact them in time. Is there any way we can help you keep this appointment?"

Patient: "I'm afraid not."

Team Member: "We have another opening at 3:30 today. Would that work for you?"

Patient: "Can't make then either."

Team Member: "I understand that emergencies pop up occasionally. Let's reschedule you. Would next Tuesday at 9 or next Thursday at 11 be better for you?"

Patient: "The Tuesday time is fine."

Team Member: "I will ink you into the schedule. Please remember that for future visits, we appreciate at least 48 hours notice of any changes. We look forward to seeing you next week."

Important Points to Consider:

1. When a cancellation call occurs, don't make it seem like it's no big deal by saying, "No problem. Give us a call when you know your schedule." Cancellations negatively affect their health and your bottom line.
2. Don't assume that it's a lost cause. You may be able to arrange for transportation or assure the patient tha a cold is no reason to cancel.
3. Don't leave the reschedule date up in the air. Get it rescheduled while the patient is still on the phone.
4. At the end of the call, remind them of your 48-hour cancellation policy.
5. End the call on a positive note.

Like many situations in your office, be respectful of your patients AND stay in control of your schedule.

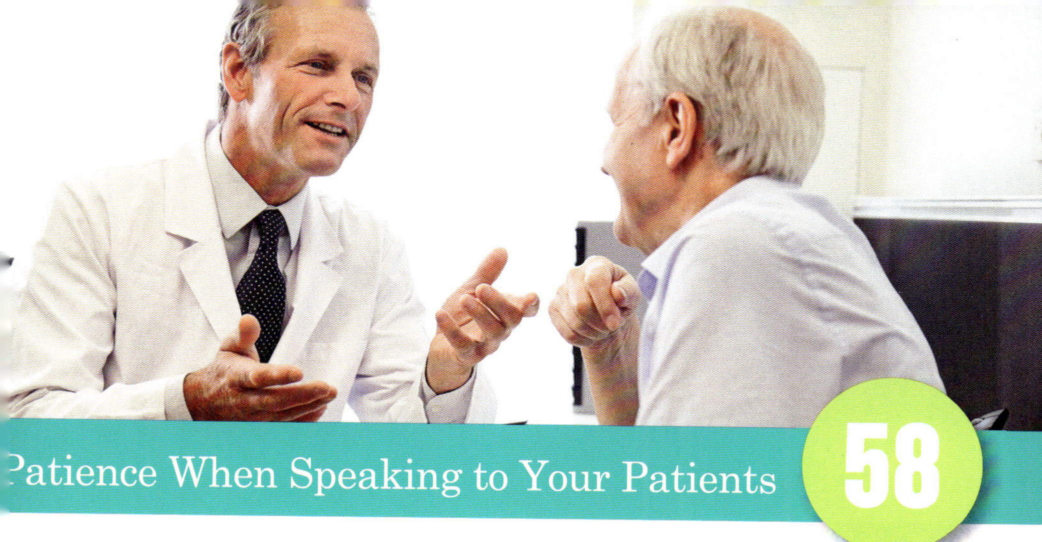

Patience When Speaking to Your Patients 58

Many of the previous tips have focused on dental practice management from an employee-employer perspective. But 's critically important we don't ignore your ractice's greatest asset: its patients.

peaking to your patients might sound easy t first. But in reality, it's far more challenging. ery often doctors are excellent clinicians – cientific and analytical – but they come up hort when it comes to their communication kills.

you're that type of dentist then this tip is for ou!

When speaking to your patients, make sure you slow down, stay friendly, and use simple, uncomplicated language. Keep the medical jargon to a minimum. Or if you do use it a bit, make sure you have a simple analogy or comparison ready to emphasize the point.

You want your patients to trust your capabilities. Just as important, though, you want to be likeable – someone they feel like they can ask any question to and get an engaging, timely response.

Practice recording mock conversations with your patients. Play them back and listen to see how you can improve. Perhaps share your findings with fellow colleagues and friends and gauge their response too.

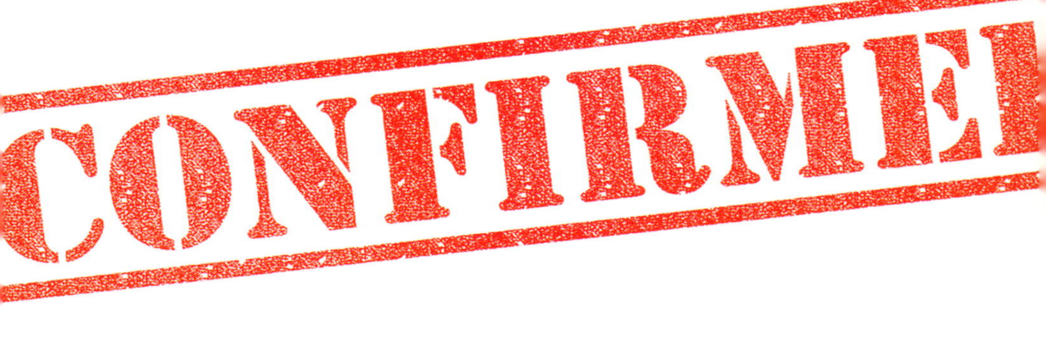

59 Confirming Visits

It's vital that you confirm visits to your office with phone calls, emails and/or text messages. Here is how the phone conversation should sound:

Team Member: "Hi, Maria. This is Debbie from Dr. Garg's office. I'm calling to verify your 11 am visit with us on Tuesday. We're looking forward to seeing you."

Patient: "I forgot I scheduled it on Tuesday. Turns out, I can't make it at 11 am."

Team Member: "Oh, no. We set aside the time just for you. Let me help you and see how we can keep your visit near that time. We have an opening on the following day at 9 am. Will that work for you?"

Patient: "That will work."

Team Member: "Excellent. Do you have a paper and pen handy?"

Patient: "I do now."

Team Member: "Great. Your visit is set for Wednesday the 5th at 9 am. I can't wait to hear about your trip to Mexico."

Three Additional Distinctions:

1. When you call, don't hand them an excuse to reschedule by saying, "You're visit is scheduled for next Tuesday at 11 am. Is that still okay with you?"
2. If you get an answering machine, leave a clear message that conveys the importance of the visit. "Hi, Maria. This is Debbie from Dr. Garg's office. I'm calling to verify your 11 am visit with us on Tuesday. We've reserved this time just for you. Please call us at 555-5555 as soon as you receive this message to verify your visit."
3. It's nice to personalize the call if you can. See the Mexico comment above.

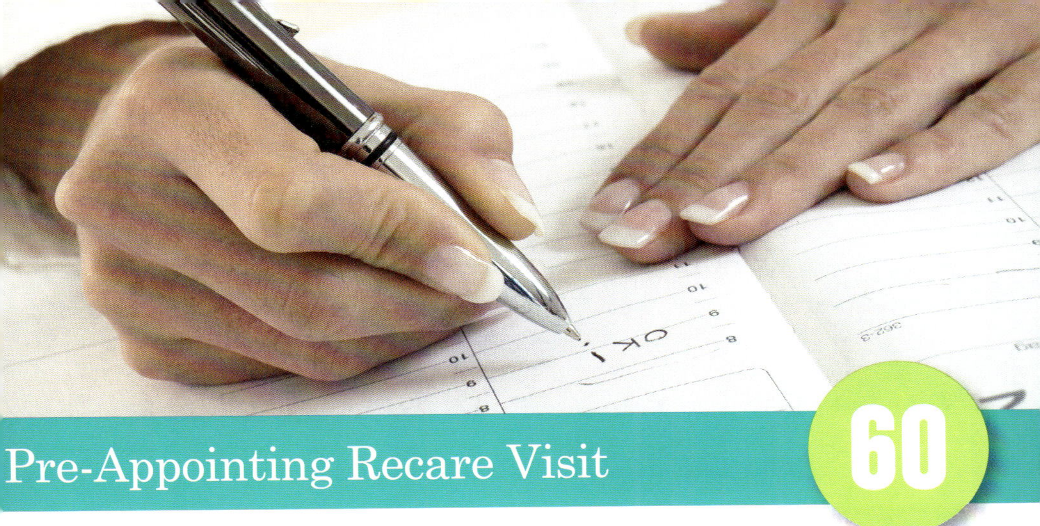

Pre-Appointing Recare Visit

60

Almost all of your hygiene patients should leave the office with their next recare visit scheduled. If they don't, it dramatically increases the odds they will delay the visit or forget it completely.

Here are three DO NOTs when it comes to making recare appointments:

- Do not ask, "Did you want to schedule your next cleaning visit now?" Many will say, "No, I'll give you a call."
- Do not say, "If you can't keep this appointment, just call us to reschedule." Or, "Give us 24 hours notice if you need to cancel this visit." When you do this, you plant the wrong idea in their minds.
- Do not give them an appointment card that says, "If this time is not convenient for you, please give us 48 hours advance notice." Do give them a card that says, "This time is reserved just for you. We look forward to seeing you."

With the above advice in mind, here is how the end of the recare visit should go:

Team Member: "Let's schedule your October cleaning and exam visit now. I know you like the first thing in the morning. Are Mondays or Tuesdays better for you?"

Patient: "I don't know my schedule for October yet. I'll give you a call in September."

Team Member: "I understand, Mrs. Jones. Our office has made a commitment to helping our patients maintain their oral health no matter how busy their schedules are. That's why we reserve a time just for you. You will receive plenty of notice. We'll send an email to you two weeks in advance and call ahead to confirm your visit."

Patient: "OK. Let's schedule it."

Team Member: "Great. Will Monday the 24th at 8 or Tuesday the 25th at 9 be better for you?"

Patient: "Tuesday works better."

Team Member: "Here's a card so you remember to write the date in your calendar."

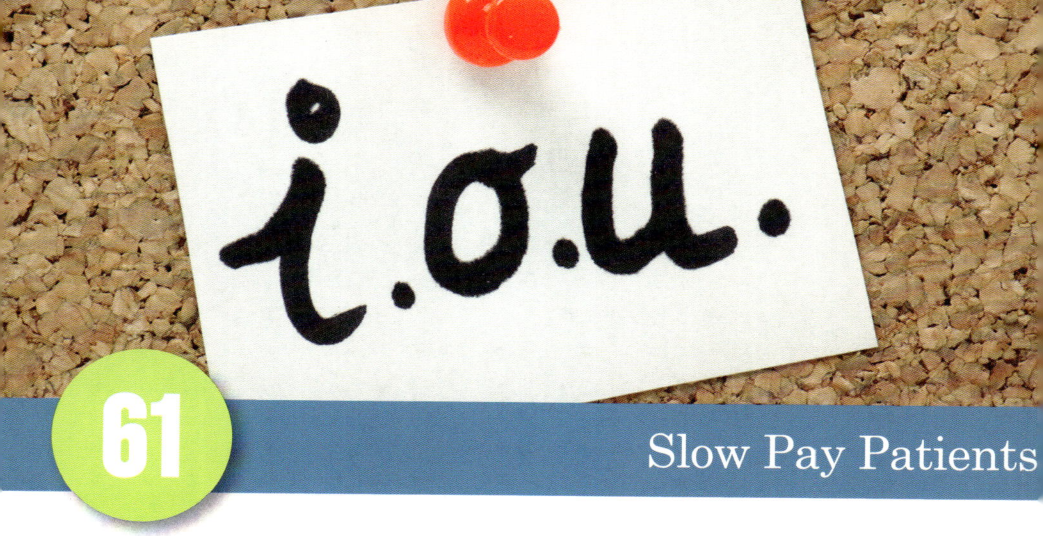

61 Slow Pay Patients

The best way to handle slow pay patients is to not extend credit in the first place. Have all your patients take care of their accounts ahead of time or on the day of service with:

- Credit or debit card
- Check
- Cash
- Third party financing

If you do end up on the hook for unpaid account balances, do the following:

- Compile a list of overdue accounts.
- Have your best administrative team member call the people on the list. The phone is a very effective tool when the responsible party answers.
- Very politely remind them of their obligation. Say, "For your convenience, we can take care of this right now over the phone with a credit card." Then be silent and wait for their response.
- If they say, "Yes," ask for their card number. A surprisingly high percentage of them will whip out the plastic.
- Then thank them for their loyalty to your practice.
- If they say, "No," explain your payment options and ask, "Which option is best for you?"
- If they say, "We can't handle that right now," say, "When will you be able to take care of your account?" Get their answer and reply, "I appreciate your willingness to take action. I will make a note of that date in our records."

Spending time collecting money is not at the top of most people's To Do Lists. But, it needs to be done on a regular basis.

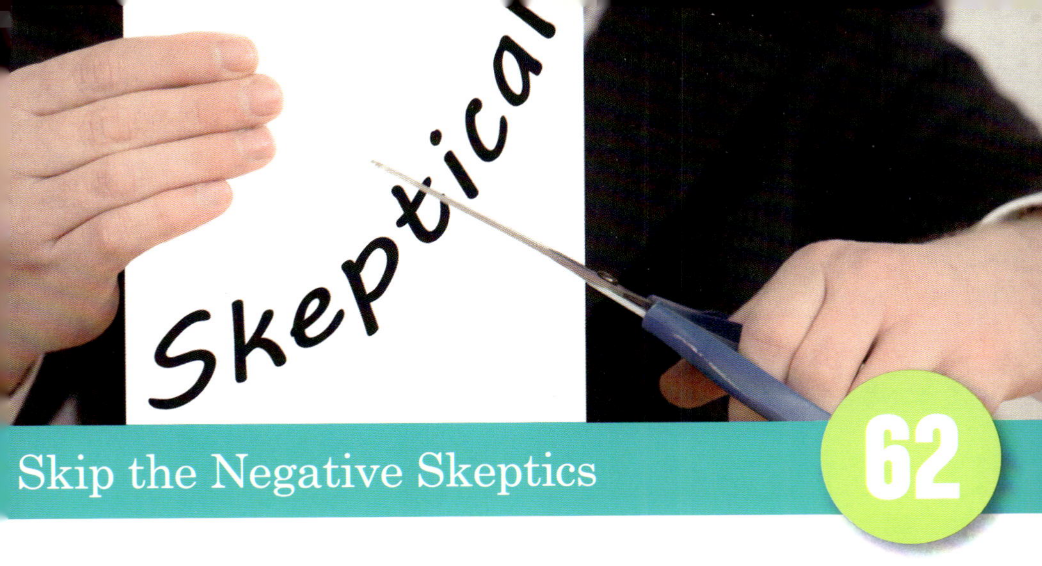

Skip the Negative Skeptics

62

Maybe you don't interact with this personality type everyday. But everyone knows a skeptic when they see one.

Skeptics are an interesting lot. It's a delicate balance they have to manage. Too much of a skeptic and you end up with a curmudgeonly naysayer. Someone who resists change and finds flaw just for the sake of doing so.

The right kind of skeptic, however, points out the pitfalls to events and the unintended consequences of ill-conceived ideas. But when they offer this critique, usually it's cushioned with a suggested alternative.

The unwelcomed skeptic doesn't have a solution. And as a matter of fact, they don't want one either. Failure is the negative skeptics fuel.

As a dental practice manager it's important to recognize the difference.

Surround yourself with positive people – men and women who aren't afraid to speak their mind when they disagree with your approach. But they must be unflinching in their efforts to offer alternative solutions to any given challenge.

Don't waste your time trying to convert a "bad" skeptic into a "good" skeptic. That energy could be better spent elsewhere – on your practice, on you patients, on you!

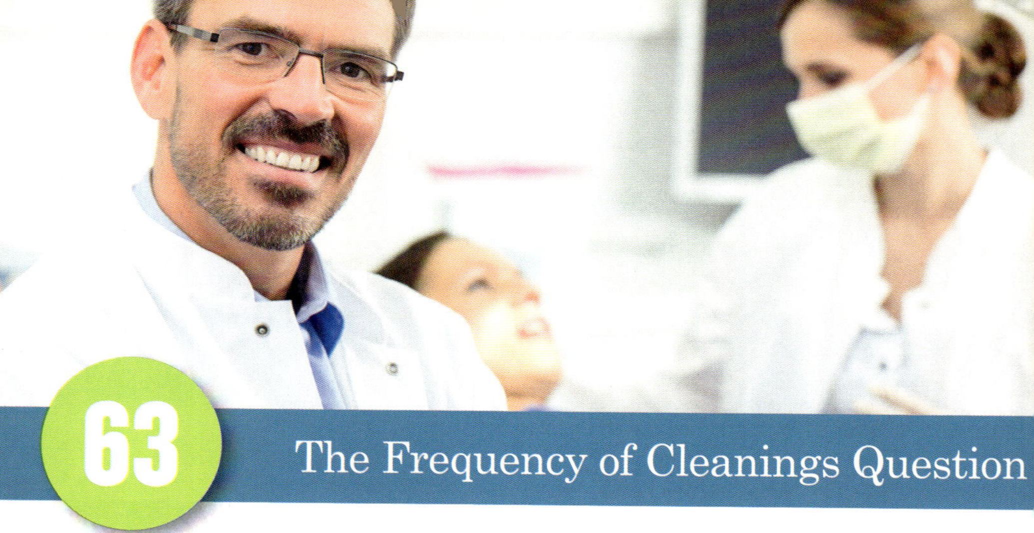

63 The Frequency of Cleanings Question

Occasionally you will get the "Why do I need to come in for cleanings so often. My insurance only pays for a cleaning every six months?" The best answers accomplish the following:

1. Never apologize for care patients need. Insurance is a method of payment, not a treatment recommendation.
2. Assure the patients that you will maximize their insurance reimbursement.
3. Explain the reasons why treatment is being recommended.

With the above three goals in mind, here is an excellent way to answer the question:

Patient: "Why do I need to come in for cleanings so often? My insurance only pays for one every six months."

Team Member: "I understand your concern. You have gum disease that requires more frequent treatment than twice a year cleanings. We always recommend care that is in your best interest. We won't compromise on that. And we will do our best to help you receive the insurance benefits you deserve."

With all the scripts you create, be sure the people using the script feel comfortable with it. If they want to make a few small wording changes, that is usually fine and will require your approval. Role playing is a vital part of effective script implementation. Have the users of the script know it so well that it rolls off their tongue without thinking about the words.

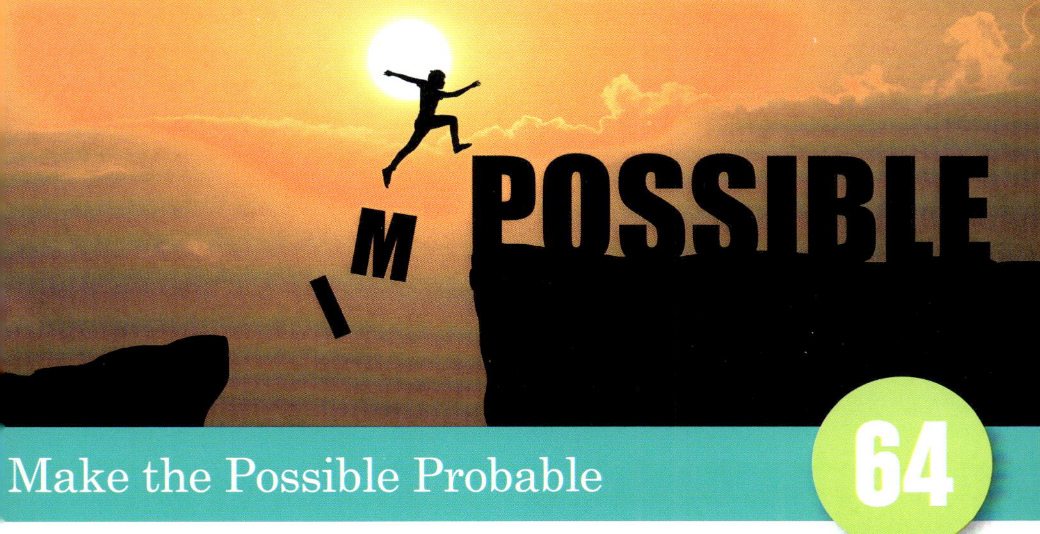

Make the Possible Probable

64

Every once in a great while all of us exceed our wildest expectations. We do more than we ever thought possible. Whether in sports, writing, hard work, humor, etc. For an instant we relish the spotlight of our own success.

Just as often, though, there's a mental recoiling that follows these bursts of incredible. The spotlight fades and we pass off our awesome as a fluke. Beginner's luck, we say. One shot in a million, we muse.

Why is it we so readily dismiss these happenings as flash-in-the-pan events? Is it a confidence issue? Is it out of laziness? Is it due to a fear of failure?

I suspect it's a combination of many factors.

The next time you experience a moment like this, don't push it away. Analyze it. Dwell on it. Make the possible probable by believing that what just occurred wasn't a fluke, but instead a window into your own true potential.

Think like that more often and I guarantee you your dental practice will begin to see a positive impact.

65 Answering Machine Message

Your answering machine message is heard more than any other message in your office. Make it a great one. Here are a few key ideas to remember when creating one:

1. Thank the patient for calling at the beginning and end of the message.
2. Remind them of your office hours.
3. Give clear instructions on how to contact the doctor if the callers have emergencies.
4. Many callers leave messages that are difficult to understand. To minimize this problem, give clear instructions on how to leave easily understood messages.
5. Do NOT say, "If you want to cancel an appointment, leave a message. Then call us if you want to reschedule." Instead, politely inform them to call you during normal business hours.
6. Be certain the person who records your answering machine message has a clear, pleasant and business-type voice.

Putting all six of the above ideas into play, here is how your answering machine message could sound:

> "Thank you for calling ABC Family Dentistry. Our office is open Monday through Thursday from 8:30 am to 4:30 pm and on Friday from 8:30 am to 1 pm. If you have a dental emergency, please call Dr. ABC on her mobile phone at 555-1212. To leave a message now, please speak slowly and clearly, spell your name and repeat your phone number. This machine does not accept scheduling changes. If you are calling about an appointment, please call back during our office hours. Thanks again for calling us."

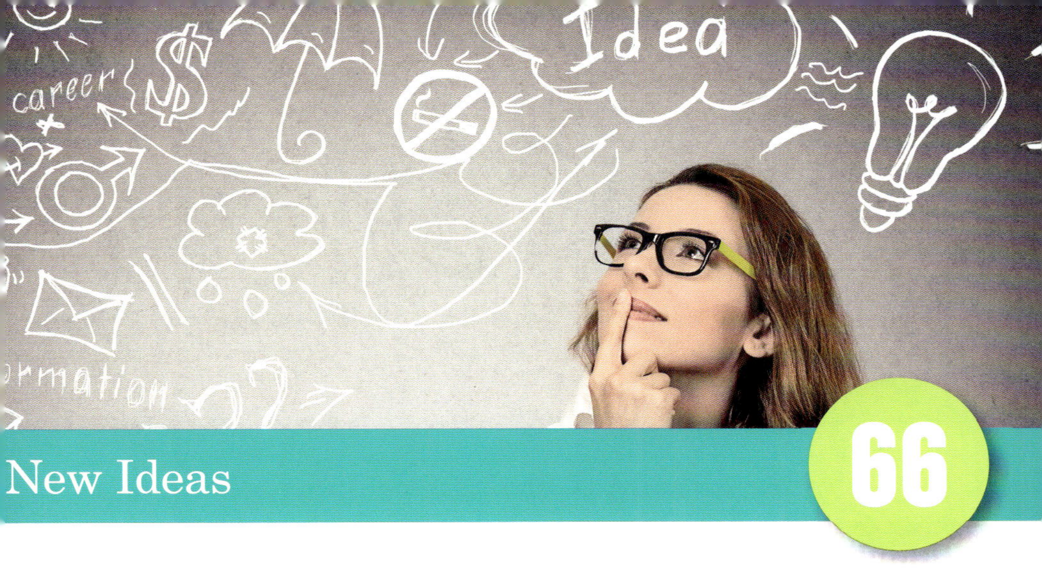

New Ideas

66

I'm bombarded with new ideas every day. Many of these new ideas are worthy of exploration and implementation. But sometimes I find myself resisting them, even though I know their potential value. I'm guessing that you face the same challenge in your personal and professional lives.

Our ability to harness the power of new ideas rests in the mental strategies we use to evaluate them, and the changes they push us to make. Let's examine those strategies now by asking some tough questions. When confronted with a new idea, do you:

- Consider the cost of switching before you consider the benefits? Is the glass half full or half empty? Half-empty thinking will stop you every time.
- Highlight the pain to a few instead of the benefits for the many? Implementing new ideas into your office may lead to decreased authority for some members of your team. It may force them to change their patterns or learn new skills. It may make them uncomfortable performing new tasks. If so, they will probably resist the change. As a leader, you must stand your ground.
- Exaggerate how good things are now in order to reduce your fear of change? Sure, things may be good now, but what about the future if you don't keep improving?
- Grab onto the rare thing that could go wrong instead of amplifying the likely thing that will go right? There is never a 100% chance of the new idea working out. Big deal. Make the change anyway.
- Focus on short-term costs instead of long-term benefits because the short-term is more vivid for you? This is an evaluation strategy I see all the time that prevents dentists from receiving the training they need to enhance their skills and improve their practices.
- Accept consistent, ongoing costs instead of swallowing a one-time expense? This kind of thinking delayed many dental offices from switching to digital radiography.
- Imagine that your competition is going to be as afraid of change as you are? Don't count on it. There are numerous new dentists and corporate dental offices out there that embrace change.

If you answered "Yes" to a few of the above questions, you may be short-circuiting your evaluation process and creating the habit of saying "No" to almost all new ideas. In the long run, that is a dangerous position to take.

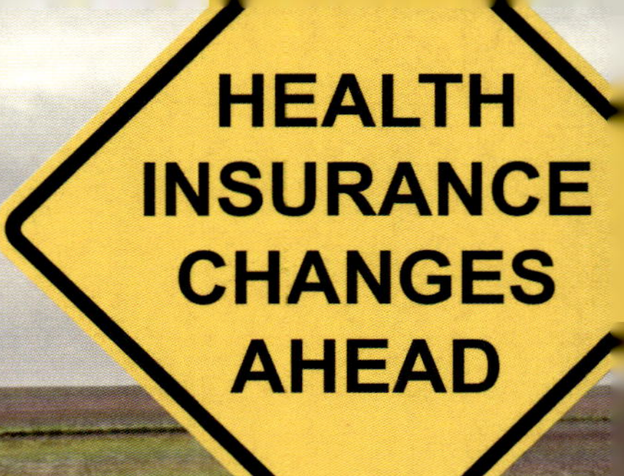

67 My Insurance Has Changed Script

Occasionally, your patients will ask, "My insurance has changed. Can you give me the name of a good dentist who is on the list?" Don't give up on keeping them. Use the following script to maximize your chances:

Patient: "My insurance has changed. Can you give me the name of a good dentist who is on the list?"

Team Member: "Thanks for letting me know of the change so we can help you. Our office has chosen to not participate in this type of reduced fee plan because we're committed to giving you the highest quality care and the best experience possible. We believe you should have the right to choose your own dental office and quality of care you receive. This type of plan doesn't allow for the best that modern dentistry has to offer.

For your protection, we've chosen not to be part of any plan that compromises the quality of care you receive. We won't recommend any dentist on the list because they have decided to accept reduced fees for their services. And with reduced fees, something has to give. Maybe it's the experience and training of the dentist and his team, or the quality of materials used, or the amount of time they spend with you. Does that make sense?"

Patient: "Sure does."

Team Member: "We can contact your insurance company to discover how your new plan really works. In some cases, you can stay with us, even though your reimbursement may be a little less." Would you like me to do that?"

Patient: "Absolutely."

Team Member: "Great. We value our relationship and hope you stay with us."

Summary

The success of this conversation rests on your ability to:

- stay positive
- educate your patients about insurance limitations
- inspire your patients to stick with you

Insurance companies want to make you look like the bad guy or gal. Don't let them do it. Shift the blame to where it belongs. It's the right thing to do.

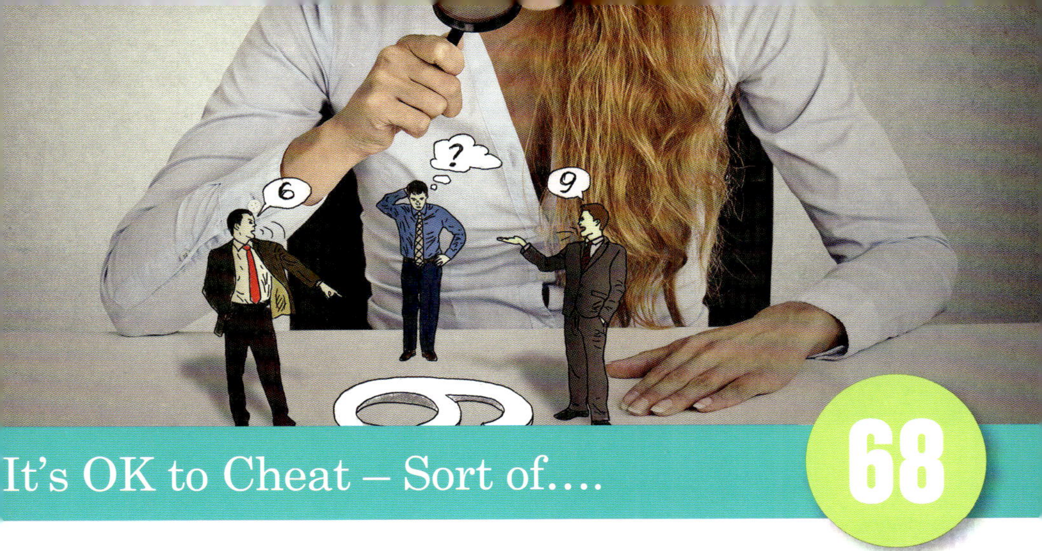

It's OK to Cheat – Sort of.... 68

OK, so maybe the above title should read, "it's OK to borrow." But chances are you wouldn't have been as motivated to read this tip! (Hint, hint, for a future tip)

In most situations stealing or cheating is morally reprehensible and outright illegal. But in many aspects of life, there exist a gray area where the line between borrowing what's considered public knowledge is a little less clear.

Playwright and social critic George Bernard Shaw put it like this: "Imitation is not just the sincerest form of flattery – it's the sincerest form of learning."

That's exactly why you're reading this book. You're gaining insight into how to improve your dental practice.

So if a colleague of yours, ideally someone outside your immediate marketing reach, is doing a better job, growing a larger practice, don't feel embarrassed to pick their brain. Be energized by the opportunity to make use of an immediate resource. Take notes, don't be afraid to ask the hard questions, and feel free to bluntly ask, "To what extent can I borrow from this idea or plan?"

It takes courage to admit someone is doing something better than you are. But I promise, you'll grow from the experience.

Is this really "cheating?" No. It's borrowing.

Feel free to borrow away!

DELIVER ON YOUR PROMISES

69 Upending Under Promise and Over Deliver

It's a clichéd expression we've come to know well: "under promise and over deliver." Translation: manage expectations by mitigating extremes.

While the expression has merit — it wouldn't be so overused if it didn't — this tip is focused on upending that logic.

Why?

Because it's not the best way to grow your dental practice. It's important to remember that big promises *do* work when you have the confidence and the quality of product to back up those assertions.

Granted, this reversal of popular expression isn't for the faint of heart. You really have to own up to the level of quality you're hoping to deliver. Otherwise, the effort could backfire drastically.

There's also an internal benefit not often considered. A staff that is properly motivated by a grand vision likely will inspire new ideas and new methods of patient engagement.

Ask yourself and your staff the following questions:

1. Are you really the best dental practice in your area? Why or why not?
2. What can you do to achieve that goal?
3. Does the quality and scope of your marketing (i.e. the promise) align with the product (i.e. the surgical care)?

So while I wouldn't dismiss "under promise and over deliver" over night, I would consider alternative promotional logic if you truly believe your talented staff can rise to the occasion and only if you believe you have the leadership skills to inspire that passion!

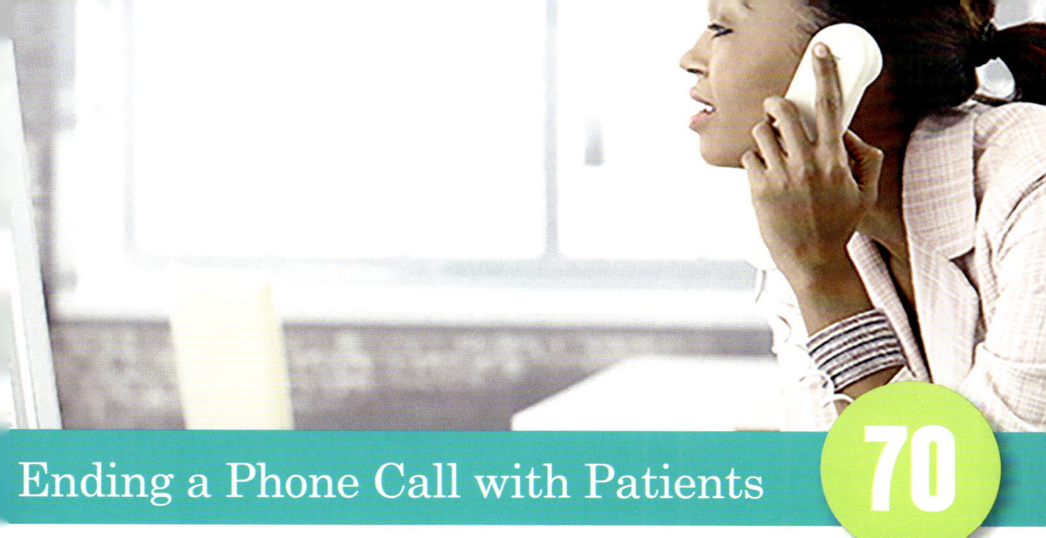

Ending a Phone Call with Patients

70

The two most important parts of patient phone calls are the beginning and the ending. The beginning sets the tone for the call and the ending leaves a lingering impression with the caller.

In previous tips, you learned the three sentence call beginning: "Thank you for calling Mayberry Dentistry. This is Darlene. I can help you."

Here is how an excellent ending should sound:

Team Member: "Is there anything else I can help you with today?"

Patient: "Not that I can think of."

Team Member: "Thank you for calling. My name is Judy. And I'll be here when you come in for your visit. If you have any questions, please call me. We look forward to seeing you."

As you can see, there are two parts to the ending:

1. Any questions? – *Sometimes patients need encouragement to ask.*
2. Look forward to seeing you. – *Set a positive expectation in the patient's mind for your next meeting.*

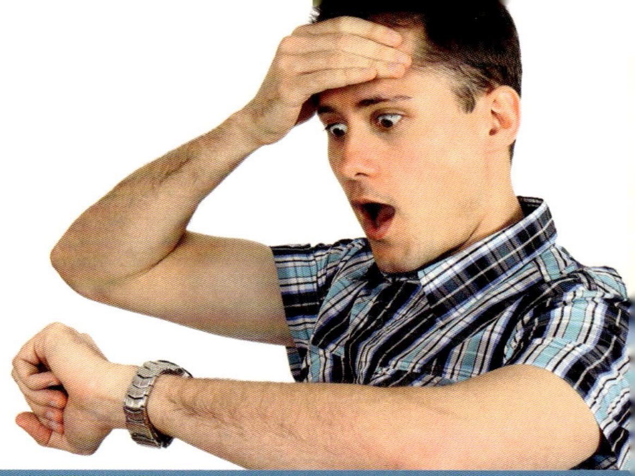

71 Chronically Late Patients

As a general life rule, you will keep getting what you put up with. Many dental practices put up with chronically late patients and no-shows. As a result, they manifest three negative results:

1. more and worse chronically late patients and no-shows
2. unnecessary stress for your team and you
3. diminished quality of care to your patients

To solve the problem, the first thing you need to do is look in the mirror. Are you chronically behind schedule? If so, correct yourself first. Then focus on them.

Do one of the following with chronically late patients:

- After an unheeded warning or two (see below), you may want give the patient a "professional care redirection" which is a nice way of saying "dismiss them from your practice."
- Put them on a special list where they can call you in the morning to see if you have any time available that day. Or you can call them in the morning to notify them of time available that day.

Here is how to say the above, "It seems like you're having difficulty keeping your appointments. Why don't you call us at 9 am on the days you're available, and we'll check our schedule to see if there is time available for you. Or we can call you in the morning when we have some time open up that day. Which way works best for you?"

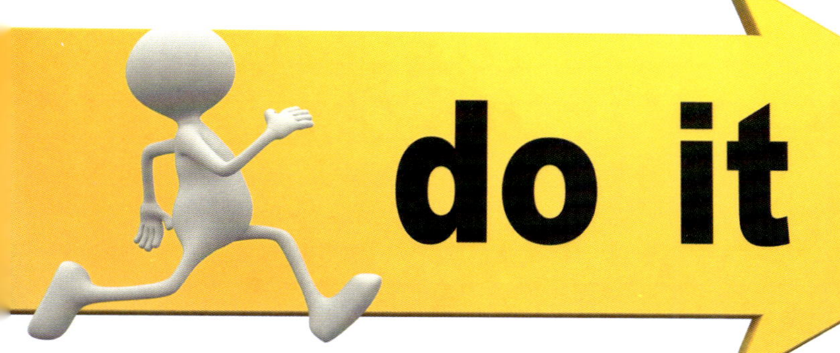

Follow Through, Don't Fall Through 72

Envisioning a new dental practice takes guts, determination, and the ability to think big. These are not trivial skills.

But it's also important to note that all of the above is entirely for free. And to a large degree, doesn't require any resources beyond your brain.

Turning ideas into action is the hard part.

So how do you follow through on your goals?

For starters, it helps if you have your goals written down. Ideally they should be organized by daily, weekly, quarterly and annual achievements. Next, decide on the metrics you want to track. For a dental office some of those metrics might include:

- How many total patients treated per month
- How many new patients added per month/quarter/year
- Feedback from surveys
- Revenue and overhead
- New procedures added and what percent of growing revenue

The most important part about envisioning your dreams is following through to ensure that they come to pass. Don't fall through the cracks of indecision, inactivity and inaction!

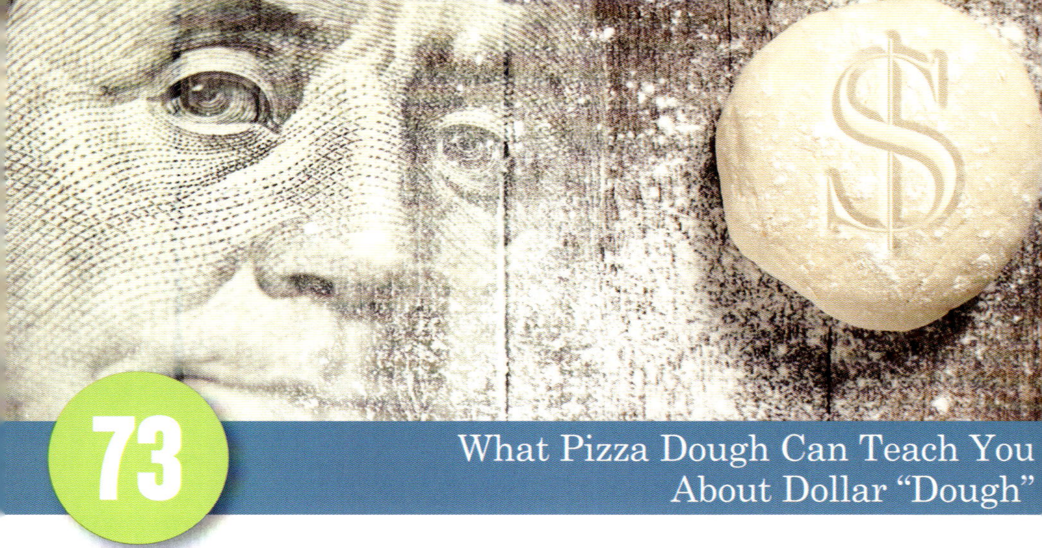

73 What Pizza Dough Can Teach You About Dollar "Dough"

Ahhh pizza, that perfect circle of eight slices of warm, crunchy (or gooey) dough, topped with a mouth-watering smorgasbord of cheese, meats, vegetables, and almost anything that your mouth and stomach desire.

Who would have thought there's a dental practice management lesson amid all this carbohydrate craziness?

Some pizzerias excel at offering variety – tantalizing toppings that could leave your head spinning. Other eateries take a different approach. They specialize in offering fewer options. Classic pizza is all you get. And the implied is assumption – with or without the Brooklyn accent – is that you're gonna love it, or else.

Dental practices would be wise to think like a pizzeria. Are you the dental practice offering all services to all people? Or are you the dental practice offering fewer, more specialized services to a narrower subset of patients?

Only you can answer what kind of dentistry you practice.

But a lesson from pizza dough might go a long way in helping you maximize another type of "bread."

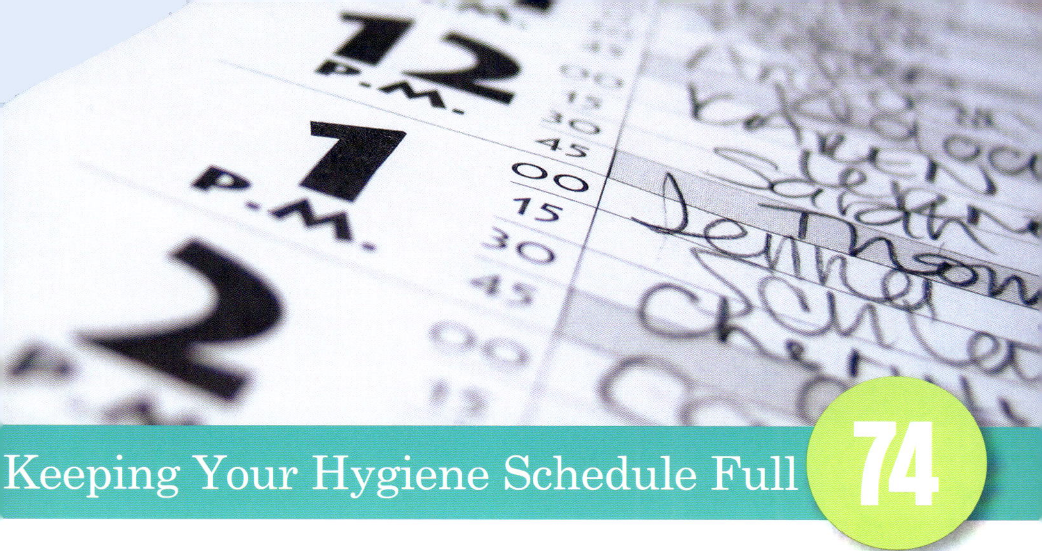

Keeping Your Hygiene Schedule Full 74

It's everybody's responsibility to keep your hygiene schedule full. Don't wait for patients to ask for their cleanings. Keep a list of patients who you know need cleanings and who have expressed desires to come in. Call them anytime you have a cancellation or no-show.

Here's an example of one way to do the above with a phone call:

Patient: "This is Carl Spackler. I lost a filling and need to see the dentist."

Team Member: "I can help you with that, Carl. Are you available tomorrow morning?

Patient: "That would work."

Team Member: "Dr. Kildaire can see you at 10 am. By the way, I see you're due for a professional cleaning as well. I'd be happy to schedule a visit with the hygienist at the same time."

Patient: "That will be great."

Four Additional Distinctions:

1. Always be thinking, "Fill the hygiene schedule. Fill the hygiene schedule."
2. Schedule hygiene visits with other visits whenever possible. It's better for them and you.
3. As patients leave their recare visits, appoint them for their next recare visit.
4. Confirm patients' hygiene visits via email and/or phone 7 days and 1 day before their appointment date.

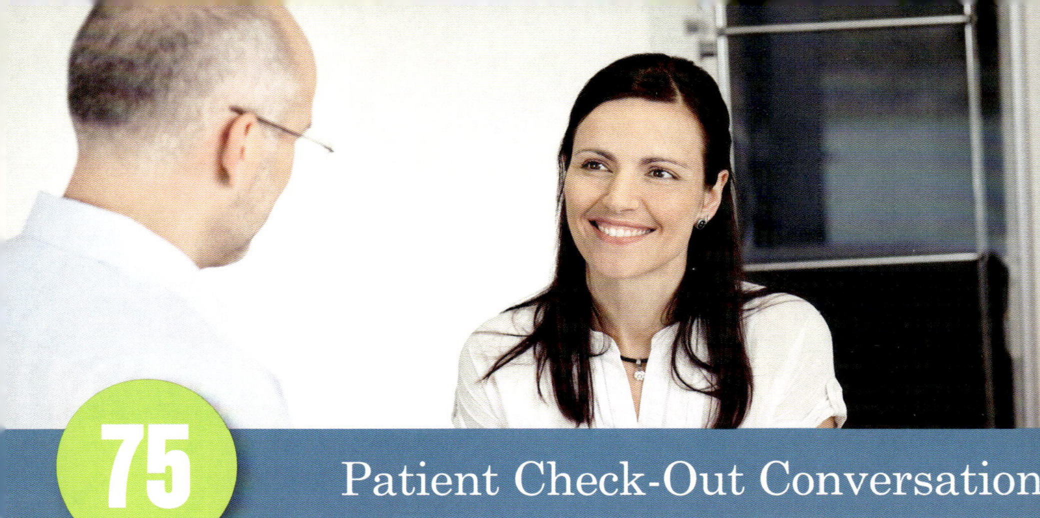

75 Patient Check-Out Conversation

The conversation you have with patients at check out accomplishes four objectives. You:

1. make sure all financial matters are handled.
2. schedule their next appointment(s) including recare visits.
3. create a positive emotional sendoff.
4. give them your business cards.

Here is how the conversation could go:

Team Member: "Tom, glad to see you're all done with your crowns. I know you were a little nervous when we got started. I hope everyone here made you feel more comfortable."

Patient: "You were great."

Team Member: "Thanks for saying that. On today's visit, you had a professional cleaning, examination, x-rays and two crowns prepared. As we discussed earlier, the total fee comes to $2,645. You chose to take care of that with Care Credit. Here's the paperwork for your signature and a copy for your records."

Patient: "That was easy."

Team Member: "Let's get you scheduled to seat your crowns in two weeks. And while we're at it, let's also schedule your next professional cleaning in six months."

Patient: "I don't have my calendar with me. I'll give you a call."

Team Member: "That's no problem at all. I will give you an appointment card to take home so you can record the time on your calendar. And we will send you an email reminder and give you a call before your visit. We'll handle everything for you."

Patient: "Sounds good."

Team Member: "Is there anything we can do next time to give you even better service?"

Patient: "No, you're fantastic!"

Team Member: "Thanks for saying that. Here are a few of our business cards. Keep one for yourself and call me if you have any questions. The other two are for family or friends who might be looking for a great dental office. Just have them give me a call."

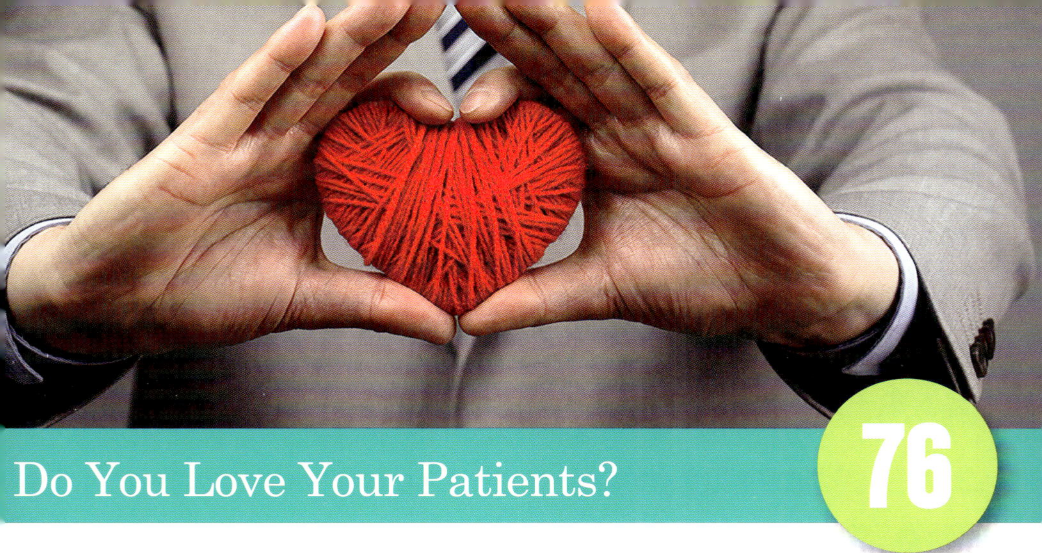

Do You Love Your Patients? 76

There are two ways dental professionals can think about loving patients:

1. "We love our patients because they pay us money." That is patients = money = love.
2. "We love our patients, and sometimes there's a transaction."

The second is very different from the first.

In the first case, patients are the means to an end… which is profit. In the second, your practice exists to serve patients. Profit is a side effect and enables you to serve at a higher level.

It's easy to argue that without compensation, there can be no service. But working to maximize the short-term profit of each transaction rarely produces long-term success. If you seek to charge above average fees for below average services, your patients will discover this, and let the world know. In a free market with plenty of information, it's very hard to succeed merely by loving the money your patients give you.

It's fascinating to note that some of the most successful organizations of our time got there by focusing obsessively on service, viewing compensation as an afterthought or a side effect. The shoe company zappos.com focuses on service to the tune of a billion dollars a year. Enterprise Car Rental is growing by leaps and bounds, not because they have better cars, but because they have noticeably better service.

As marketing gets more and more expensive, it turns out that loving your patients for the right reason is the best shortcut to trust, which leads to all the other benefits that a growing dental practice seeks.

Your patients can tell the difference. And they vote with their loyalty to your practice in dozens of ways. So love them… regularly… for all the right reasons.

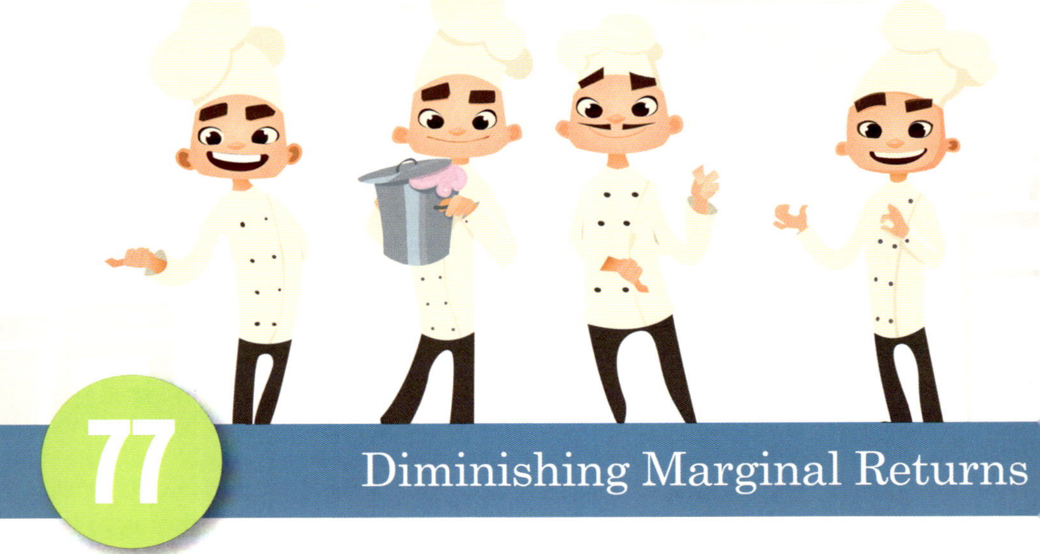

77 Diminishing Marginal Returns

Diminishing marginal returns is an economic principle taught in most high school intro to econ courses. And for good reason. It's one of the most important.

The textbook definition goes like this: "the law affirms that the addition of a larger amount of one factor of production, while all others remain constant, identified by the Latin term "ceteris paribus," inevitably yields decreased per-unit incremental returns."

Simple translation: Too many cooks spoil the broth.

Adding new staff, expanding your skill set, or purchasing expensive CBCT scanners and the like, all sound like great ideas at first. And they are. In moderation. Attempt to do too much too quickly and the value you receive from each addition will begin to diminish.

Don't overcomplicate what's already working. Enhance your practice slowly. Add new staff, but don't overwhelm existing employees or give them too little to do. Purchase that CBCT scanner. But only after other aspects of your practice are running smoothly and you have the time to commit to learning how the machine works and how to read the scans taken.

Keep your "dental broth" brewing beautifully and remember the law of diminishing marginal returns.

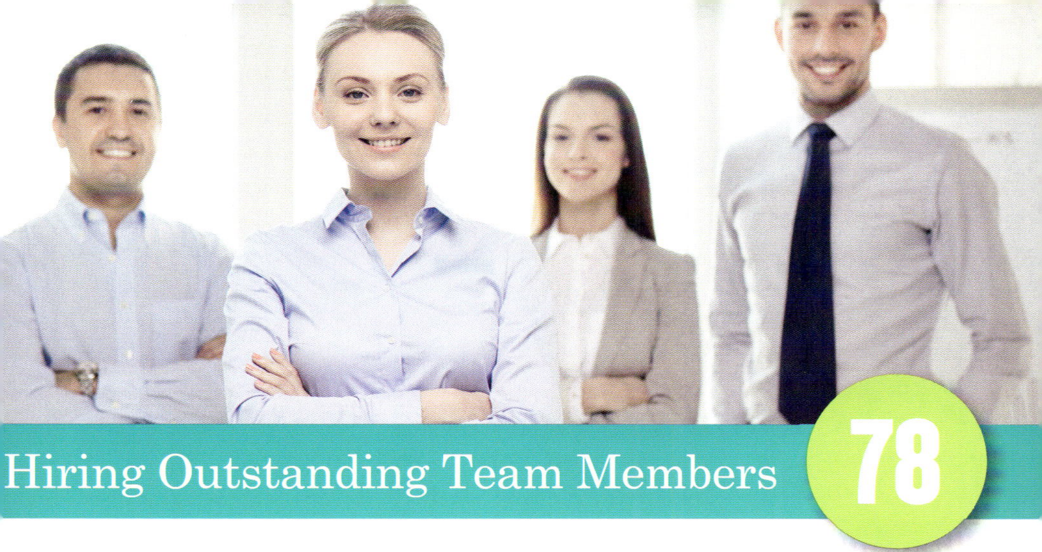

Hiring Outstanding Team Members 78

You graduated dental school knowing how to cut a mean MOD. But nobody ever said anything about how to hire outstanding team members. The difference between comfortable and downright wealthy is in large part dependent upon your ability to hire superstar team members.

The hiring process is as complex as the exacting steps necessary to prep and seat eight veneers. Make an error during any step along the way, and the result can be disastrous.

There's no fool-proof system for hiring the best team members. A smart fool will figure out a way to beat almost any system. But there is one step in the hiring system that will help minimize the chance that your existing team will dislike the new person. Have you ever hired a new team member that you thought was great, but your existing team didn't like? How well did that go?

Have Your Existing Team Take Ownership of the Hiring Decision

Here's one simple step that will ensure your team becomes invested in the success of your new team member. After evaluating the candidates' ability to write email responses to a blind email address. And after listening to how they speak on the phone by them leaving voice mails telling you more about themselves. But before inviting them to the office for an in-person interview, **HAVE TWO TEAM MEMBERS CONDUCT PHONE INTERVIEWS WITH THE CANDIDATES.**

Independently, each of the two team members chats informally with the candidates by phone. Each team member has the right to eliminate any applicant. In order for the candidates to attend an in-person interview, they must have the approval of both existing team members who spoke with them.

Although there is no one step which will ensure success in the hiring process, doing the above will go a long way toward building a harmonious team of happy people who work together and pull in the same direction. These folks are happy to help each other, happy to help your patients, and happy to assist you in creating the practice of your dreams.

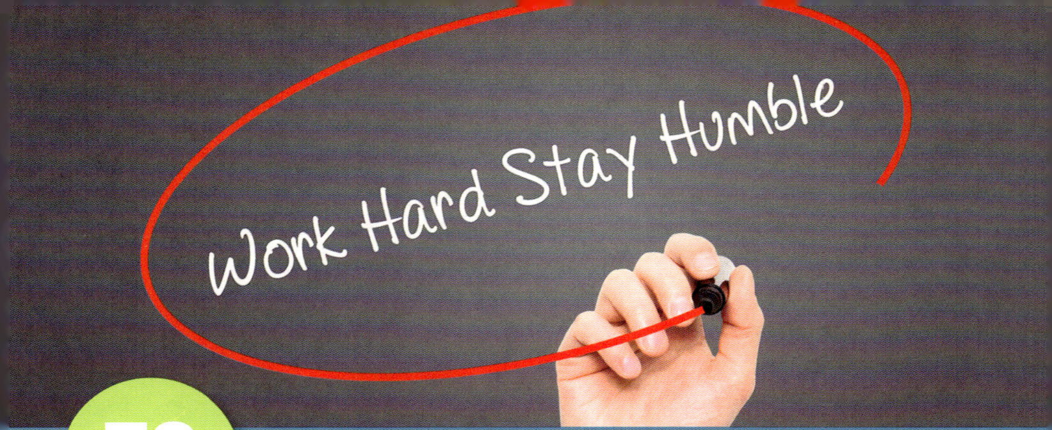

79 A Little Humility Helps…

For all the time and money you spend investing in your dental practice and plan for its growth, it's easy to forget the importance of humility.

The brutal truth is that as with most people in life, we are all replaceable. If suddenly your dental practice didn't exist tomorrow, 99.9 percent of your patients would seek alternative treatment. In short, you're really not that special.

Sorry to burst your bubble, but it's true.

This doesn't mean you shouldn't chase perfection (to borrow from football coaching great Vince Lombardi). It means that as great as we think we are, there's always room for improvement. And that no matter how good we get, someone still will likely do it better. If not now, then eventually.

Humility helps. Embrace it!

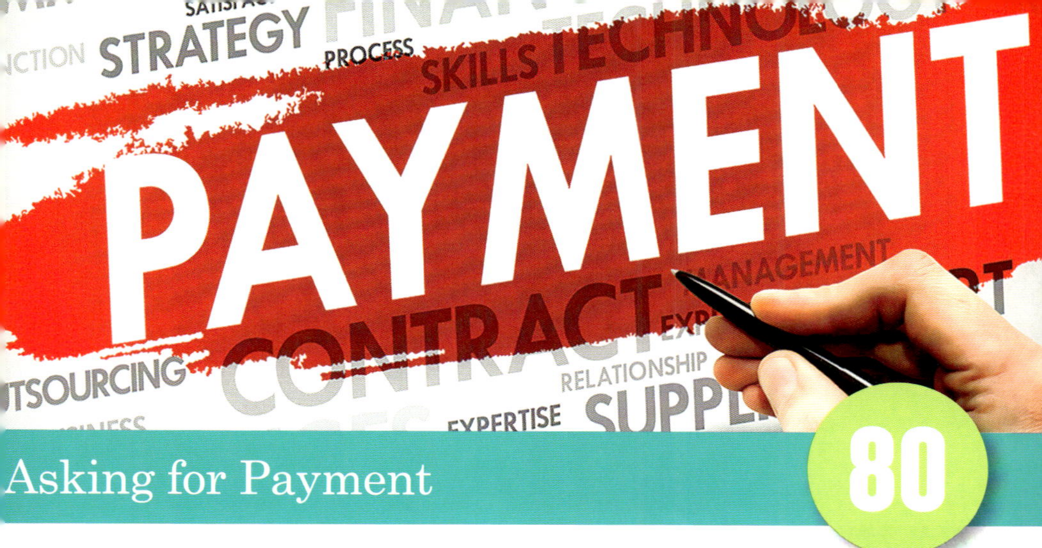

Asking for Payment

80

Asking for payment of fees at the time of service can be difficult for some team members. To make it easier, have the request memorized and keep it short and sweet. Here are three ways to do it:

1. "The fee for your treatment today is $220. You can pay that by cash, check or credit card before you leave. Which way is best for you?"
2. "We offer a 5% courtesy for payment in full today with cash, check or credit card. This makes your payment $209. Which payment method is best for you?"
3. "We ask that you pay your estimated insurance co-payment of $500 at your visit today. Will that payment be comfortable for you?"

Additional distinctions about asking for payment:

- Have payment discussions before treatment, not afterwards.
- Don't say, "The fee is $300. OK?" This question doesn't state a clear payment arrangement or explain when the payment is due.
- Don't say you "need" or "require" a payment. Ask that patients pay at the visit. This means the same thing and sounds more respectful.
- Always end the conversation with a polite call to action. The three call to actions above were, "Which way is best for you?", "Which payment method is best for you?" and "Will that payment be comfortable for you?"
- Effective payment arrangements by your business team before treatment will virtually put an end to patients receiving treatment and then saying, "I didn't know I had to pay today." Or "I forgot my checkbook."

Receiving payment at the time of service is better for you because now you don't have to bill or chase people down. And it's better for them. It's one less bill for them to worry about.

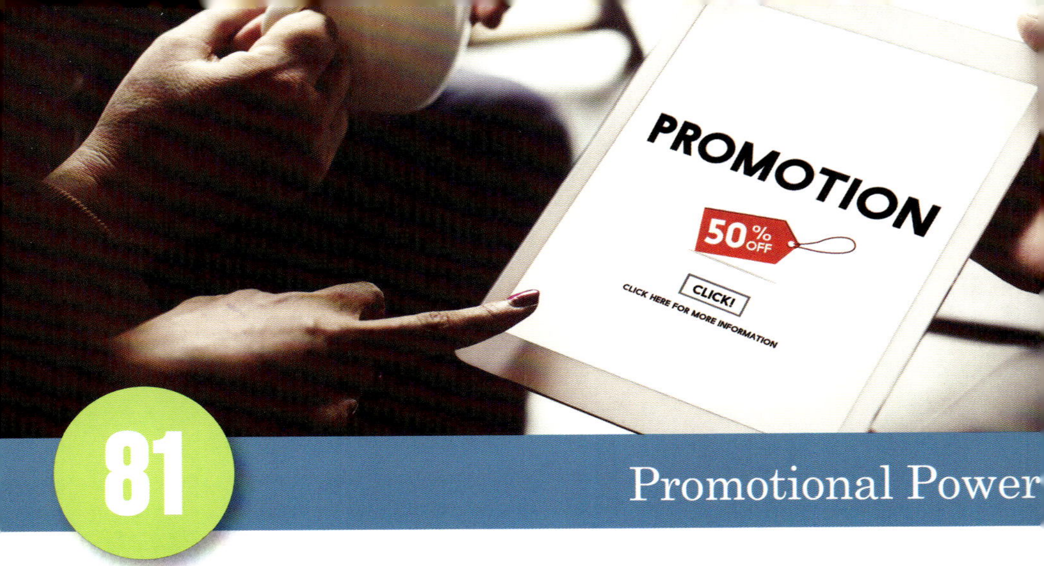

81 Promotional Power

Turn on the radio, watch TV, or check out your favorite websites of your favorite brands what do you see? Discounts. Bargains. Deals of the day. And a bevy of special promotions.

But sometimes all-day discounts can backfire.

Think back to 2012 and J.C. Penney's failed "fair and square" marketing strategy. By doing away with inflated prices in order to make discounts look more appealing, the company tried a more honest approach of lower prices all the time.

But the perception of the deal proved too powerful to ignore. Even if prices under the new J.C. Penney plan had been better, the perceived discounts (due to the dropping of fake prices) rapidly eroded.

Not long after this realization, customers began jumping ship. By the fourth quarter of that year, same-store sales dropped 32 percent!

As a dental practice manager, it's important to take stock of your prices too. Don't be afraid to offer a periodic promotion – tailored to a specific day, season, time of year, or even to particular patients who have spent X dollars with your clinic in the last several months.

Learn from the failed J.C. Penney model, though, and never forget that the perception of a discount is often just as or more important than the actual cost of care.

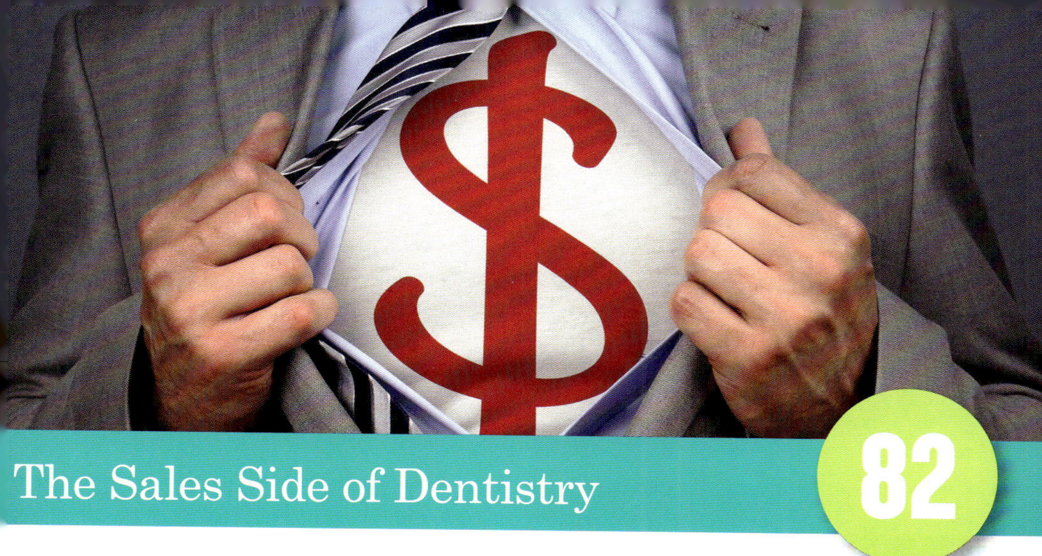

The Sales Side of Dentistry

82

You may not employ actual sales staff on your dental team and that's perfectly OK.

But you would be wise to encourage your team to think like salespeople at least some of the time. Actually, if you didn't promote your business and the treatment you offer, you wouldn't be in business very long.

It's a tough skill to master. Especially when dentists, office managers, dental assistants and hygienists aren't trained sales professionals, it's easy for them to think sales people are too pushy for the medical profession.

If "salesman" and "saleswoman" are descriptors that sound too strong, remember that as medical professionals, you're all in the business of giving patients the best care possible. As a dentist you've gone to school, you've earned a valuable degree. You have the responsibility to promote treatments that will improve your patients' lives. Like it or not, that is a type of sale.

So how do you encourage your dental staff to think like salespeople? Well for starters, I recommend attending seminars and talks given by marketing experts on exactly these topics. Investigate what continuing education opportunities are available in your area and encourage your staff to attend. Perhaps incentivize their attendance further through additional paid time off, a subsidized lunch, whatever perk you can think of in order to boost attendance.

Second, I would augment these marketing and sales courses with your own in-office refreshers. Schedule a relaxed lunch where you can all discuss what you've learned. Maybe even role play between prospective patients and front office staff. Review scenarios and encourage "curveballs" be thrown to make the mock conversations more difficult, but also more realistic.

Don't resist the fact that to some extent we're all in sales. Whether you're promoting your dental practice, or going on a job interview, or trying to land your first date, self-promotion is the name of the game.

83 Social Media Savvy Dentistry

With 974 million Twitter users and 1.65 billion people on Facebook — nearly a quarter of the world's population — it makes sense, then, that businesses join the social media bandwagon too.

But just because you're on social media doesn't mean you know how to use it right.

Too often brands think of social media as just another platform to post a digital billboard of sorts. This goes for dentists too. Just mentioning a discount or new deal in a tweet or a Facebook post isn't really maximizing the tools at hand.

As the term implies, social media is all about being social. That means engaging your customers. In a dental framework that could mean posting stories and articles related to dentistry and dental trends. It could also mean writing your own. Anything that generates a conversation about oral health and the advances in imaging or treatment planning could be beneficial.

What about sending daily or weekly tweets related to insurance company reimbursement? This is a perennial topic for dental patients.

Showing your patients that you care about them in the office and out of the office, carries an emotional premium. And it's a small effort that demonstrates your office cares just a little more than the competition.

Sometimes, in the competitive race to be the best, that little bit of added effort is all you need to truly stand out.

So tweet away and Facebook post until your heart's content. Just make sure you do it right!

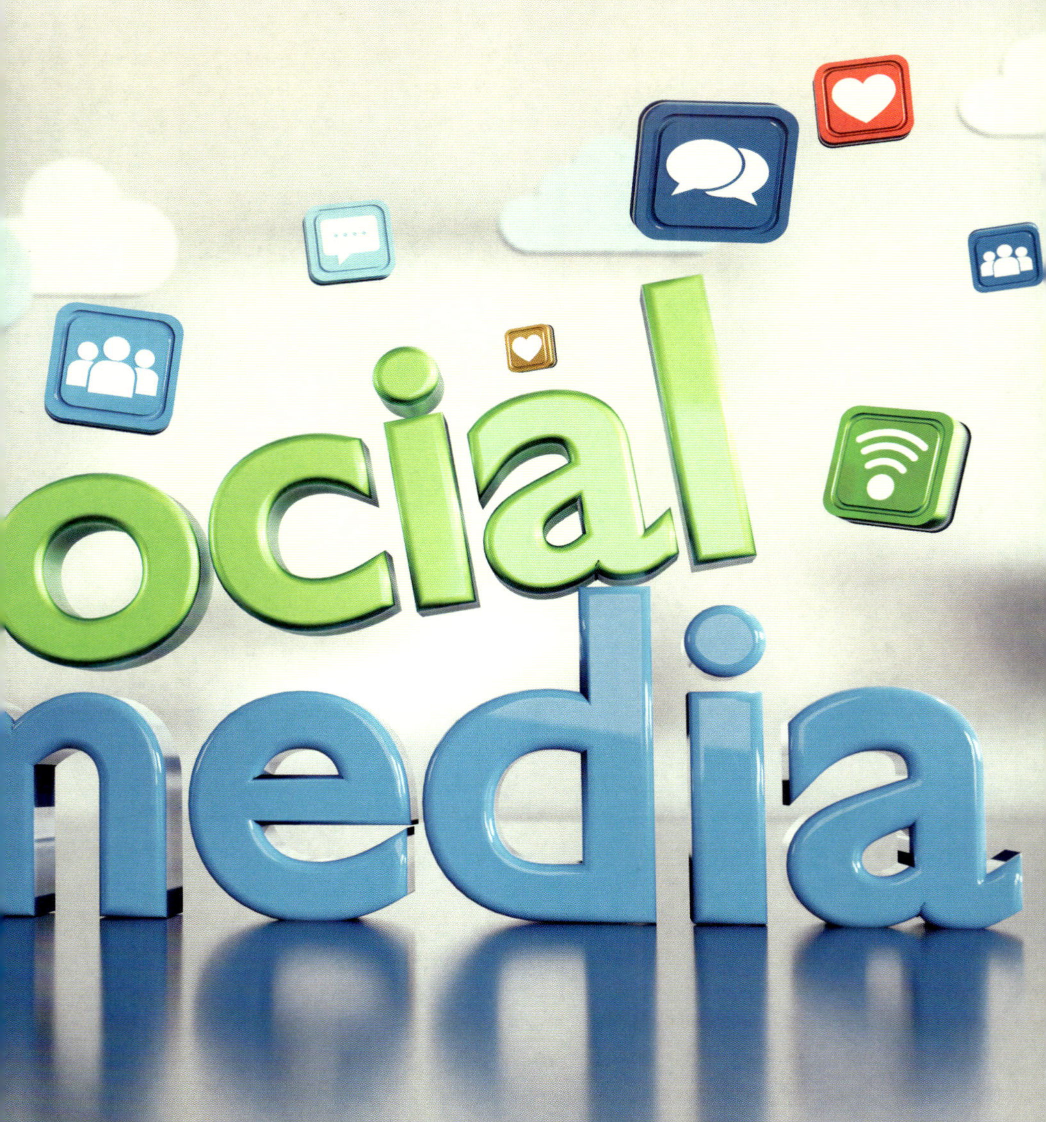
ocial
edia

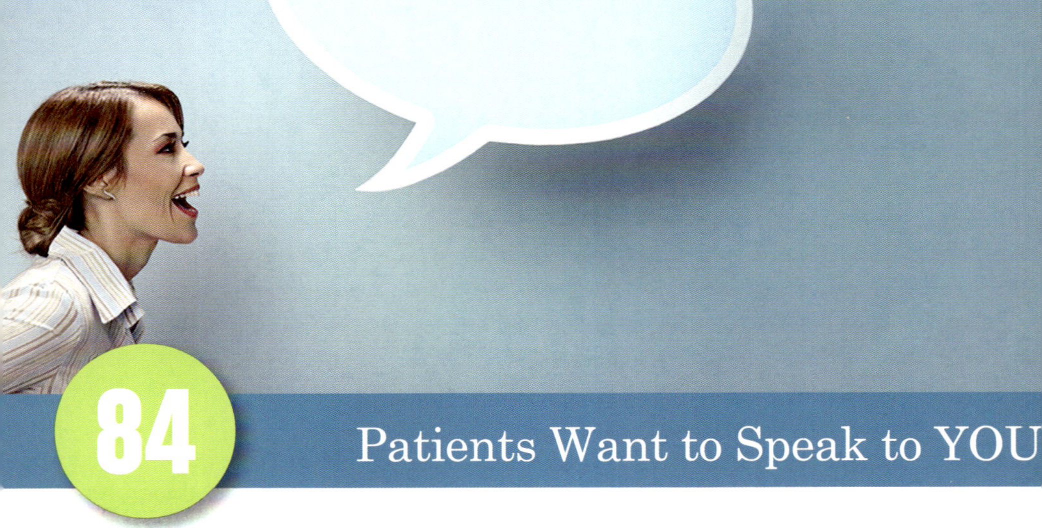

84 Patients Want to Speak to YOU

You know the patients I'm talking about. The ones who demand to speak with you about issues the front office personnel can and should handle. Here is one way your team can effectively handle these patients:

Patient: "I don't like the way you answered my question. I want to speak to the doctor, now."

Team Member: "I understand that you'd like to speak with the doctor. However, he is here to provide you with exceptional dentistry. I'm here to help you with any concerns or questions you have."

Patient: "So I can't speak to the doctor?"

Team Member: "As I mentioned, it's my responsibility to handle all patient concerns about financial and service issues. The doctor depends on me to take care of these matters so that he can devote all his time to your dental needs."

Most patients who ask to speak with you really don't need to. And your team members can almost always handle these situations better than you. But you must empower them to do so. Schedule a meeting with your team and agree on how to handle these calls. Give your team a script to use and have them role-play it.

Occasionally, it might be best for your team members to discuss the patient's concerns with you. In these situations, they should avoid telling the patient, "I need to check with the doctor." Have them say something less specific like, "Let me check on that and call you back." This way, your involvement, if any, is kept confidential from the patient.

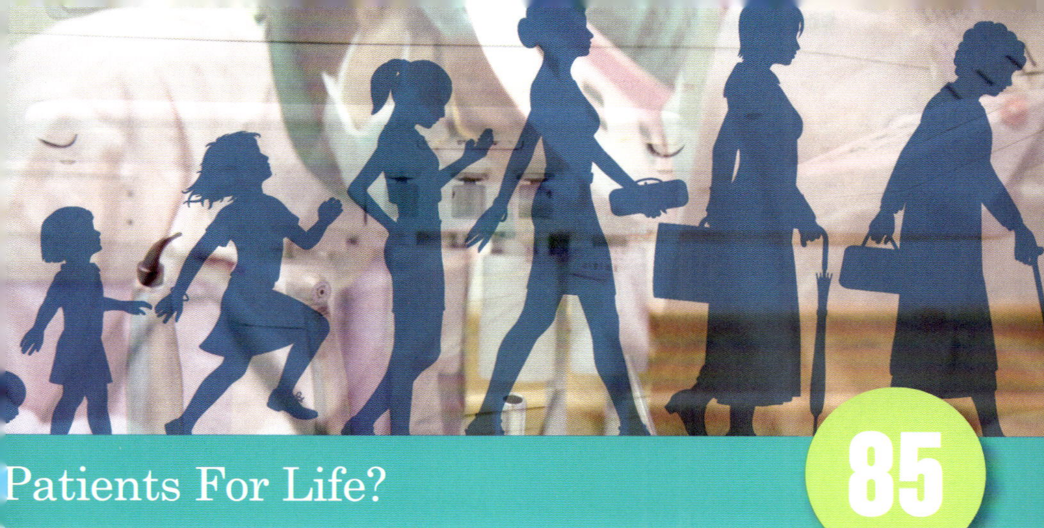

85 Patients For Life?

Imagine this scenario. You're 35 years old. You've been out of dental school for several years. You've worked in a dental practice. And now you're in a position to buy your own. Congratulations! What's the first thing you do? Is it:

A) Research all the practices up for sale in your area and begin making phone calls and sending email/Linkedin outreach?

B) Start thinking about the type of practice you'd like to be and the type of staff that fits your mold?

C) Evaluate your financial goals and your current liquidity. How much can you really invest in this new venture with X thousands of dollars in dental school bills outstanding?

D) Envision your ideal patient, brainstorming how you can keep them patients for life.

E) Look to take on a partner because you know the operation you plan to run will quickly grow too large to be managed by one person

OK. So maybe the title of this tip makes the correct answer a bit obvious. But I strongly believe that patients come first. Dentists are in the business of healing people and transforming lives. If we didn't put patients first, we wouldn't be the healers we claim to be. And without patients, we wouldn't have a dental practice.

So no matter which way you slice it, patients – not the staff, not the equipment, not the software, and not even the dentist – are the most important. The question is, how do you make them patients for life?

First, you have to believe this is possible. You have to believe in yourself that you can cultivate a professional, yet personal relationship with people spanning the next 30-40 years. It's about being genuine, about being caring, and about going out of your way to walk in your patients' shoes.

For lifer patients aren't for lifers because of discounts and deals. They stick with you because they like you. So be likeable. Be approachable. Be honest, but don't be callous.

Once you've begun building a dental practice with patients you can expect to keep for life, only then should you begin addressing the other answer choices listed above.

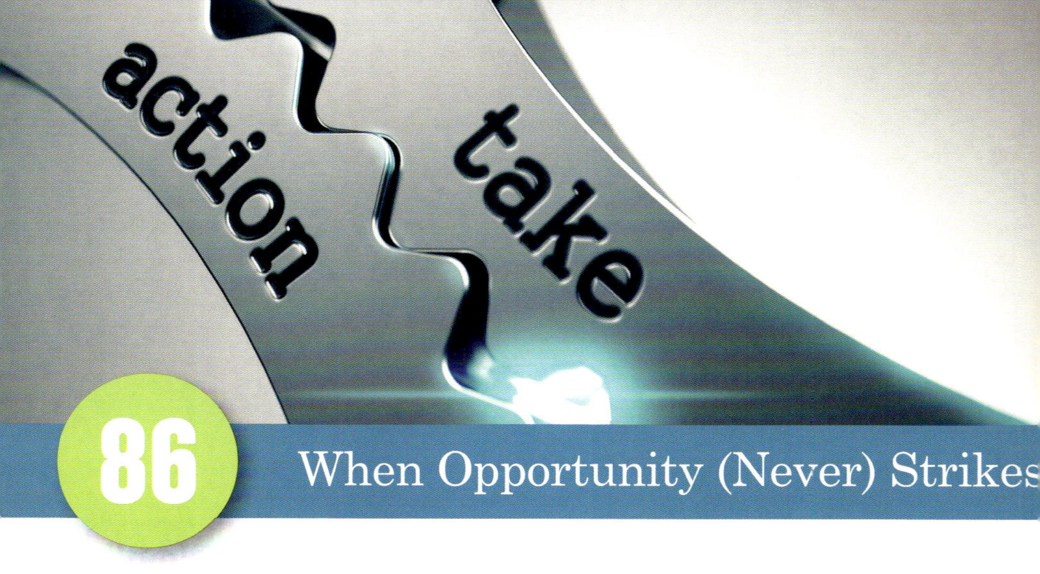

86 When Opportunity (Never) Strikes

When it comes to intellectuals there are three kinds of people: doers, thinkers, and executers.

The doers and thinkers are great people, but they have a problem. Sometimes the doers do without thinking and the thinkers dream up the incredible, but fail to action what they envision.

The executers are the perfect hybrid. These are the people who think about their actions and follow through on their plans.

The question is, what kind of a dentist are you?!

Don't make excuses for why something can't be done. Give reasons for why something must be done!

Some people wait for opportunity to strike. Others strike out for new opportunities. Be the dentist that capitalizes on those lucky breaks!

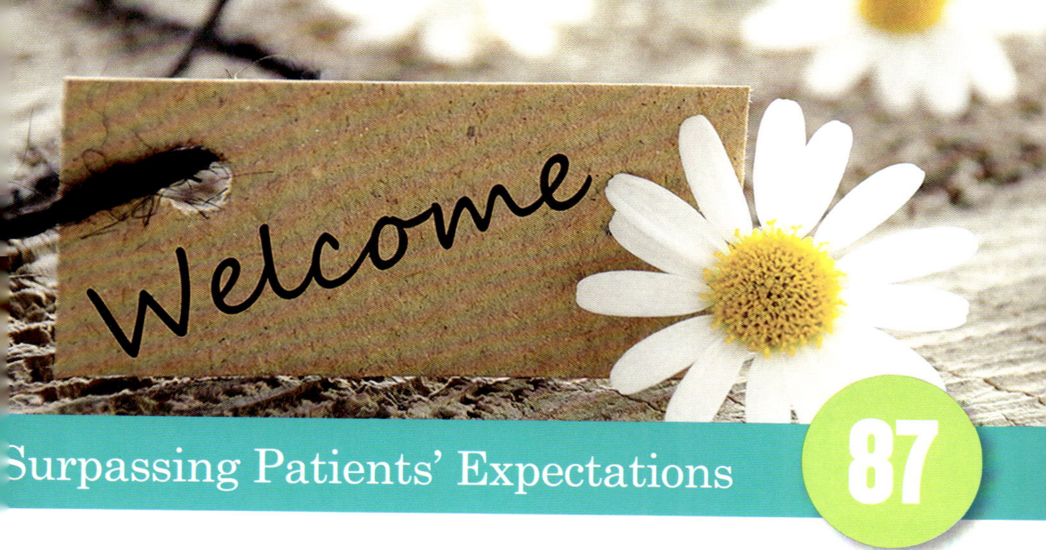

Surpassing Patients' Expectations 87

ne of the most important conversations your team can have with patients is the one that occurs when the patient walks ı the door. It sets the tone for the entire isit including discussions you may have oncerning case acceptance and financial rrangements. Most dental offices I visit say omething along the lines of, "Welcome to ur office, Mrs. Henry." That's not bad, but it ould be so much better. Here's how to do it:

ew patients

n excellent greeting for your new patients , "Hello, Mrs. Henry. I'm Alejandra. We poke on the phone the other day. Welcome our office. We're glad you're here."

ırrent Patients

n excellent greeting for current patients is, Welcome back to our office, Mrs. Henry. /e're glad you're here."

lditional Distinctions

1. When possible, go into the reception area to greet new patients.
2. Offer a handshake, even to children.
3. If you're on the phone or helping another patient, acknowledge the patient by smiling and waving.
4. With new patients, offer to help them fill out the forms. Say, "If you have any questions about the forms, just wave at me. I'm here to help you."
5. When escorting new patients to a treatment room, give them a brief tour of the office and ask, "Is there anything I can do to help make your visit more comfortable?"

Make Their Experiences Better Than Their Expectations

Patients have expectations when they enter a dental office… especially for the first time. These expectations are primarily determined by their experiences in other professional offices. When the experiences you provide are a little bit (and sometimes a lot) better than what they're expecting, you create delighted patients. This is way better than satisfied patients. Delighted patients can't help themselves. They feel compelled to tell others how wonderful you are. And this free advertising is the best kind you can have.

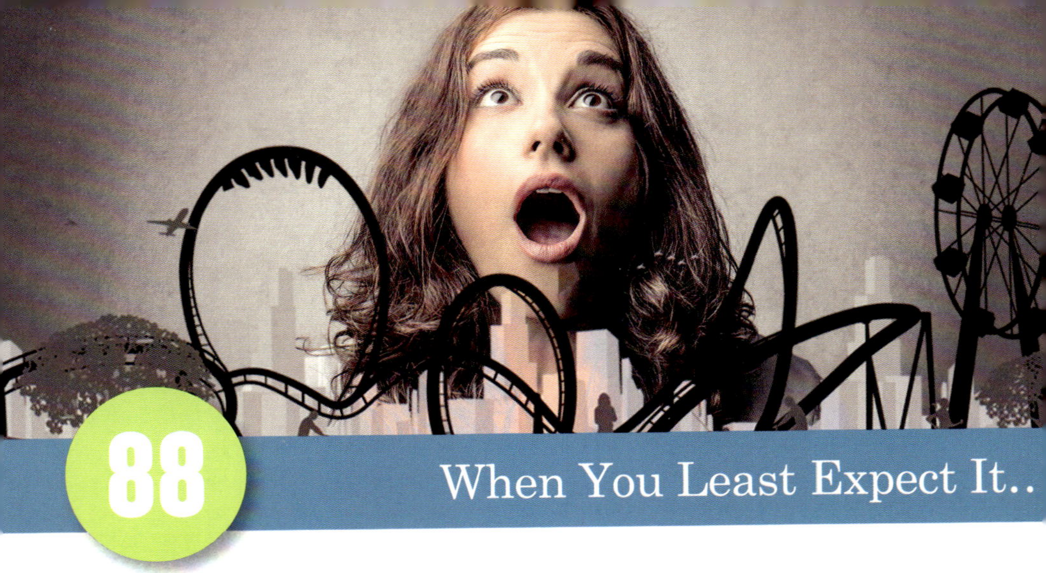

88 When You Least Expect It..

Sometimes you gotta go with your gut. Put down all the marketing tips books, ignore what your best friend says, and forget about reading market trends. (Just remember to read this tip.)

It's important to consider that many of history's greatest breakthroughs have been of the impromptu kind. And on those occasions very often an invention or different way of doing something was roundly criticized.

- In 1966 *Time Magazine* declared remote shopping would be a failure. Why? Because women like to get out of the house and handle the merchandise.
- How about in 1904 when a French professor noted that "airplanes are interesting toys but of no military value."
- And my personal favorite: "There is no reason anyone would want a computer in their home." This brainy quote comes from Ken Olson, founder of Equipment Corporation in 1977.

In fairness, Olson's comments came at a tim when computers were still bulky room-sized affairs. But that's just the point. It takes a special person to pursue their dreams even when naysayers line up to criticize what's possible.

Will your dental practice herald a new treatment planning methodology? Will you b able to provide remote dental care via drone Probably not. But hey, what do I know?! Success happens when you least expect it. So grab hold and enjoy the ride!

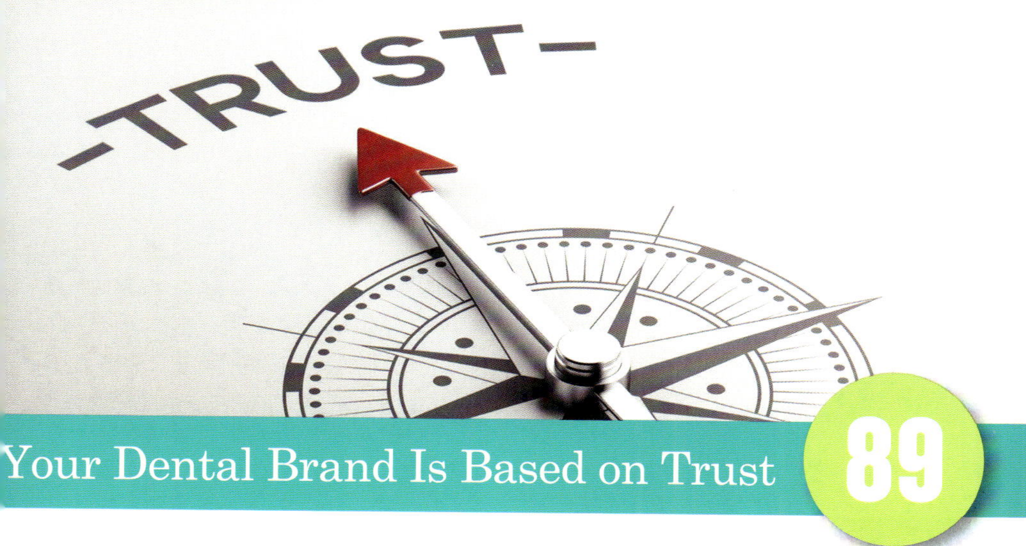

89 Your Dental Brand Is Based on Trust

Your dental practice extracts enormous value from the relationships you have with patients, team members and suppliers. Your dental brand is based on trust. Trust is vitally important, but it's not free. **To gain and maintain it, you will need to do things that are difficult.**

Your brand is also a series of promises you make to people. And you must keep every promise… especially the little ones. And when you do, trust will be earned.

So, it's vitally important to not say things like:

- "I just couldn't get back to you."
- "I'm sorry, but my hands are tied."
- "Well, because you complained, just this one time. But don't ask us to do it again."
- "I know Sue told you that, but she doesn't work here anymore."
- "Sure, we used to do that, but too many people took advantage of us, and we can't do it for you."
- "That's our practice policy."
- And most common of all, silence.

If you do any of the above or their closely related trust-busting cousins, patients will trust you less. And the diminished trust damages them and you.

It's easy to convince yourself into believing that you can be trusted at the same time you take short-term profits and cut corners when it suits you. Alas, that's not going to happen. Trust can be expensive. And building and keeping trust is worth it.

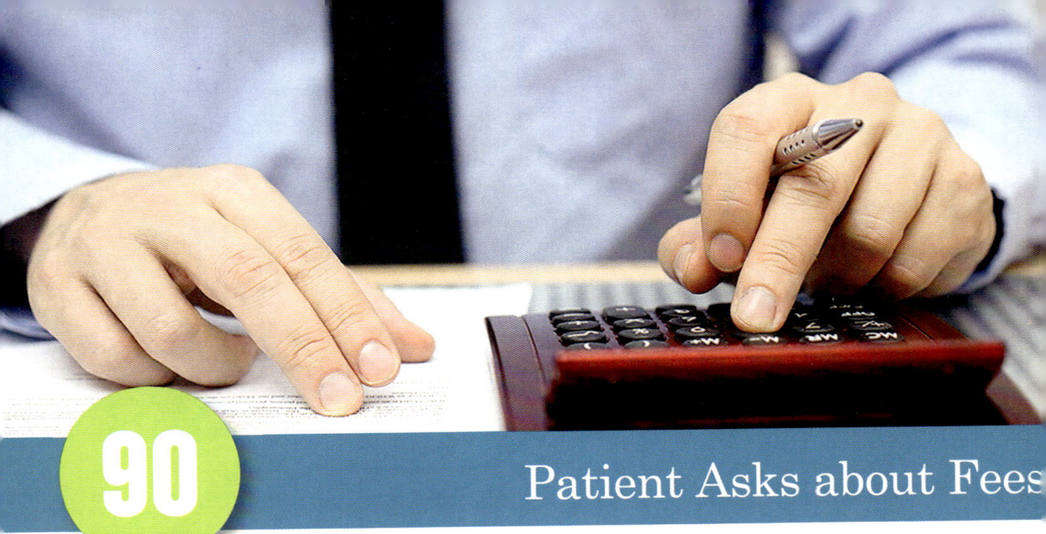

90 Patient Asks about Fees

Patients occasionally ask fee-related questions such as, "How much will those two crowns cost?" I have seen two approaches work when answering that question:

1. Team members refer the question to a financial coordinator by saying, "That's a good question. I'll go get Lorraine, our financial coordinator. She's an expert on fees and financing. She'll be happy to help you."
2. Team member or doctor quotes the fee if they know it by saying, "If the tooth doesn't need a build-up, our fee per crown is $1,100. I'll go get Lorraine, our financial coordinator. She's an expert on fees and financing. She'll be happy to answer all your questions and make the arrangements."

I know. I know. We've all heard it a thousand times that only financial coordinators should quote fees. That may be the safest way, but it's not always the best way. I believe that dentists and all team members need to be prepared to answer most questions about fees. Then refer the financial arrangements part of the process to the financial coordinator. Always remember that just quoting a fee to an agreeing patient does not make it a payment agreement. Only your financial coordinators should do that.

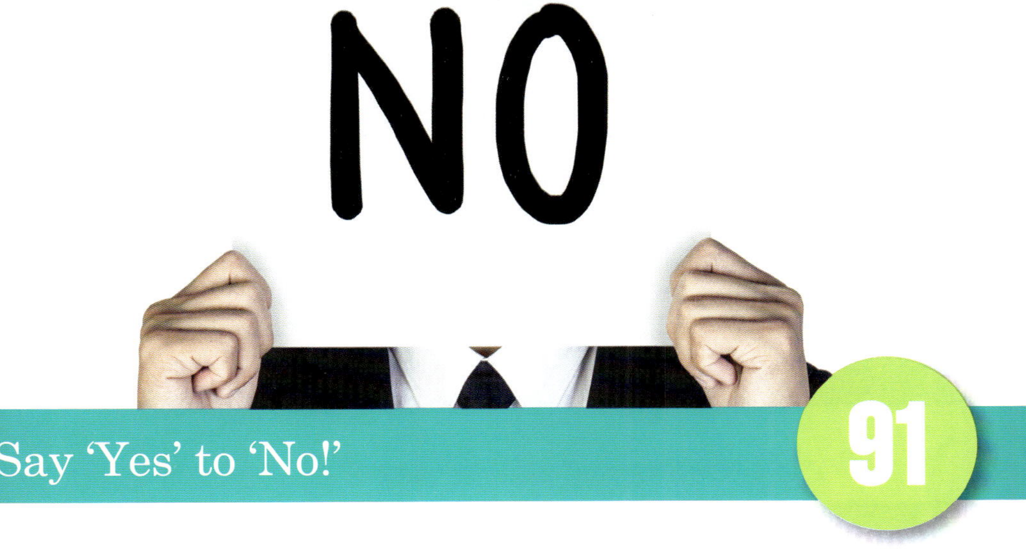

Say 'Yes' to 'No!' 91

No. It's a simple, two-letter word used to express dissent, denial, or refusal.

So common is it, that 'no' is among the first words babies learn to say, usually around word number 7 – ahead of cat, nana, bye, and duck.

But for a word that has such negative, limiting connotations, it's important to remember how valuable it can be.

Saying 'no' means saying 'yes' to something else. The key is to say 'yes' to the right things. When it comes to managing a successful dental practice, say 'yes' to:

- Growth
- Pleasant patients
- A can-do, positive attitude
- Networking opportunities

Admittedly, this tip is unlikely to upend your world. But taking a step back and learning to embrace the power of 'no,' could be the first step in the type of dental practice you envision.

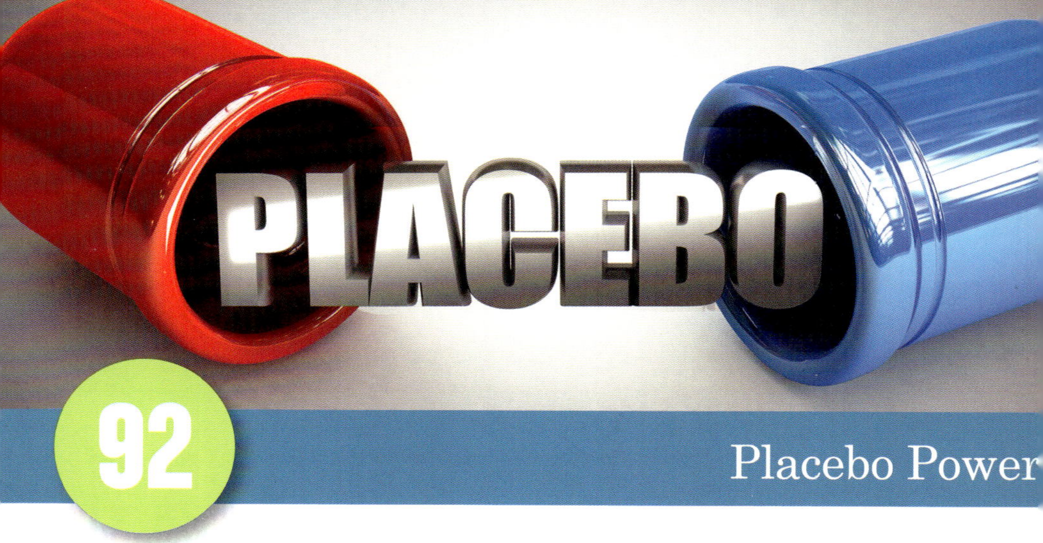

92 Placebo Power

You may not believe this, but your patients want to have a positive dental experience – even if they're fearful of the outcome.

The placebo effect is a well-studied medical phenomenon. People who take a fake pill, but believe in its effectiveness, will nevertheless feel improvement.

Your dental practice can operate under a similar logic. Update your waiting room; add an assortment of new periodicals; make free Wi-Fi available and include informative videos on TVs or on tablets for your patients to review. Combined with a friendly and efficient staff, your patients' fears will begin to subside. They will begin to anticipate a more positive visit.

It's a fact. Happier patients make better patients. Surgical risk is reduced, as are postoperative complications. And the happier they are the more likely they will be to recommend your services to someone else.

So don't dismiss the power of placebo. It could very well transform your life.

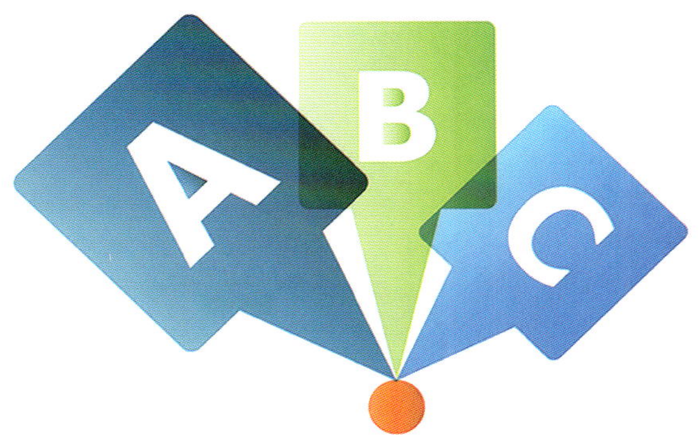

The Patient is Overwhelmed

93

It's always an uncomfortable conversation… for you and them. A patient has just received a comprehensive treatment plan with a correspondingly hefty fee. They are shocked with both. Here's an excellent way to handle the situation.

Patient – "I can't believe how much work I need done and how much it's going to cost. I guess I shouldn't have waited so long to come in."

Financial Coordinator – "We're glad you're here now. I know that you feel a little overwhelmed. I just want you to know that I'll be with you through every step of your treatment. Do you have any other questions for the doctor or me about the recommended treatment?"

Patient – "Not really. It's the finances I'm worried about. How can I pay for all this?"

Financial Coordinator – "Some of our patients have the same concern and the same question, so I understand where you're coming from. We have several payment options to help you. Let's see which one works best for you."

Additional Distinctions

- Always align with the patient by communicating, "I know how you feel."
- Patients are often intimidated to ask the doctor follow-up questions about recommended care. Offer to clarify the treatment plan before discussing financial arrangements. This will significantly increase your case acceptance percentage.
- Never prejudge the patient's ability to pay for care. Assuming from their appearance that they're too young, too old or too poor to afford comprehensive dentistry is a big mistake.
- There is a school of thought that says when people send an emotional message that it is an act of kindness or a cry for help. The patient message described above is definitely a cry for help. Respond to their cry with understanding and kindness. It is the right thing to do.

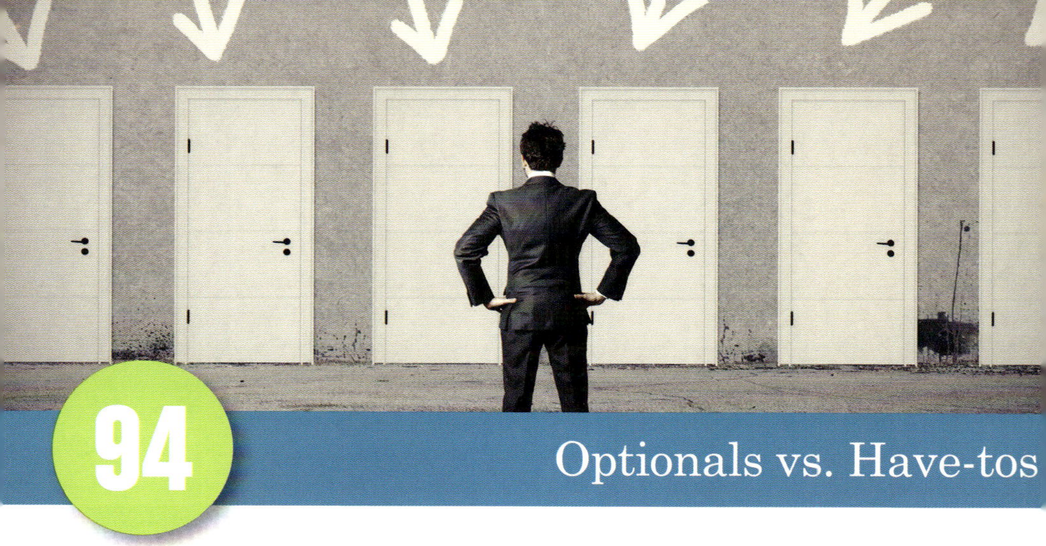

94 Optionals vs. Have-tos

Perhaps it's a simplistic way to look at life, but there are "optionals" and "have-tos." Maybe it's even something a first grade teacher would say to their students about homework.

Optionals are up to the individual's discretion, while have-tos are obligatory.

But you'd be surprised how often people confuse these opposites. We forget to look on the bright side and remember that so much of our life is within our control. We have choice. We have free will. Yes, at some level, we all have to pay the bills. We all have to eat and drink in order to live. And in order to have a successful dental practice, we have to keep our staff and our patients happy.

How we achieve these goals is entirely up to us.

When you think about it like that, doesn't it inspire you for the greatness that's yet to come? Celebrate the optionals in life, because when you get down to it, the have-tos is a pretty short list and what's on it is boring and obvious.

Enjoy the freedom to grow your dental practice any way you see fit.

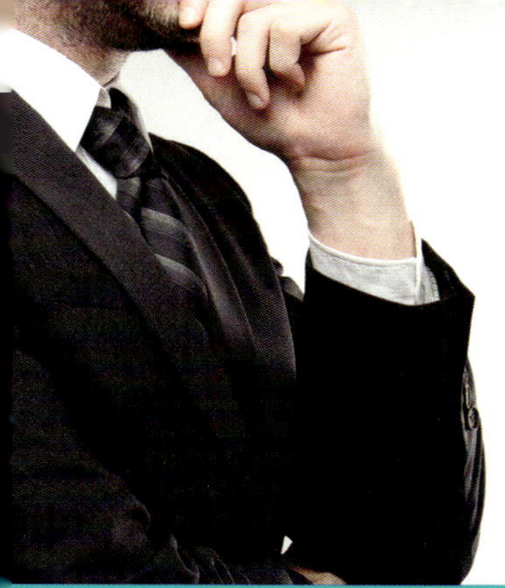

Other People's Choices About You

In the last tip, I discussed the choices you make in life. Your happiness, fulfillment and success in life are partially due to these choices. But most dentists don't realize that other people's choices about them are equally important.

- Do people choose to come to your dental office?
- Do patients choose to accept your treatment plans?
- Do people choose to refer family and friends to your practice?
- Do your children choose to follow your advice?
- Do people choose to be your friend?

The choices others make about you are heavily influenced by your ability to create three types of connections:

1. Liking – People tend to do business with people they like.
2. Rapport – People prefer to hang around others with whom they feel a sense of commonality.
3. Trust – People are more apt to accept the advice of professionals they trust.

In the next three tips, I will show you how to create each of these three types of connections. This is vitally important to your emotional and financial success because you can be the most skilled clinical dentist in the world and do all of the technically hard dental procedures extremely well. But if you haven't mastered the soft skills of dentistry (liking, rapport and trust) you will never reach your full potential.

It all begins with you taking responsibility for communicating and treating others in ways that create their reactions to you. It's all too easy to blame them for their "ignorant" choices. Don't fall into that trap.

I hope you find all of the Tips valuable to your practice and life. The next three Tips on liking, trust and rapport may be the most important ones I've written.

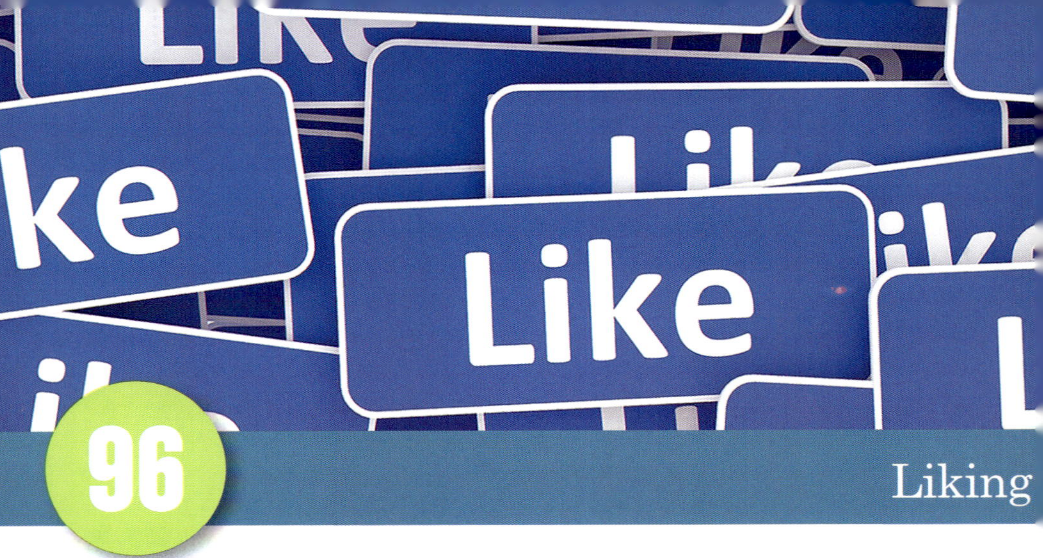

96 Liking

It's a fact of life. People tend to do business with people they like. Think of the person who cuts or styles your hair. Do you like the person? The answer is very probably, "Yes." It's possible you don't like the person, but are a customer anyway because of the person's fantastic skills. This rarely occurs because people don't usually do business with people they don't like.

Here are five ways to increase your likeability quotient:

1. Give patients sincere compliments and ask follow-up questions. Examples are: "Love your shoes. Where did you get them?" and "You're a fun person? Did you grow up in a funny family?"
2. Thank your patients for their loyalty. Say often, "We appreciate you as a patient. Thanks for coming to our office."
3. Smile. A smile is the universal signal for, "I like you."
4. Use positive words and phrases such as:
   - "Absolutely."
   - "Yes."
   - "I'll take personal responsibility to make sure that gets done."
   - "It would be my pleasure." Every time I ask our computer man to do something, he replies, "It would be my pleasure." It's a very nice touch... and unexpected.
5. Show interest in your patients' personal lives. Use the Sandwich Technique:
   - Talk about personal things first. This could be children, where they live, the patient who referred them, sports, a vacation or a big event.
   - Do your dentistry.
   - Talk about personal things just before they leave.

Delivering high-quality clinical dentistry is a vital component of your practice's success. And when you pile high levels of likeability on top of it, you have a powerful combo that will attract numerous high-quality patients to your practice.

Rapport

97

Rapport is created by a feeling of commonality with people – a sense that you're "on the same wavelength" or "in sync." Gain rapport with your patients by taking the following steps:

1. Discover things you have in common with patients through short conversations. Use the information you discover or a team member discovered on the first phone call. When in doubt, talk about the weather or some local news. Enter the personal information about each patient in the Notes page in your practice management system.
2. Leave your clinical or business area, wander out and talk with folks in the reception area. They will love it.
3. Sit or stand at their eye level.
4. Mirror their posture.
5. Take off your mask and loupes. You're a living, breathing human. Not the Lone Ranger.
6. Match their conversational style. Talk softly and slowly if they are. Their brains will unconsciously whisper, "Ah, a friend." The same goes for your extroverted patients who talk loudly and quickly and use a lot of hand gestures. Be extroverted with them.
7. Enter their worlds. If a patient is struggling justifying the cost of treatment enter their worlds by saying, "It looks like you're wondering if the investment is going to be worth it. Do you mind if I tell you what I hear from other patients?" Or if they seem perplexed with their replacement options, enter their worlds and say, "You seem a little confused with the three options you have for replacing those teeth. Would you like me to clarify your choices?"
8. Do little unexpected things for people. Little unexpected actions have more rapport building than big expected action. Some dental examples are:
   - Make care calls the day of any procedure that required an anesthetic
   - Write thank you notes to men on Father's Day
   - Present women a flower on Valentine's Day
   - Write a few thank you notes every day

Rapport is a soft, fuzzy thing. And the soft, fuzzy things in a dental practice can be the hardest to achieve. Make the effort. It will pay off for everyone.

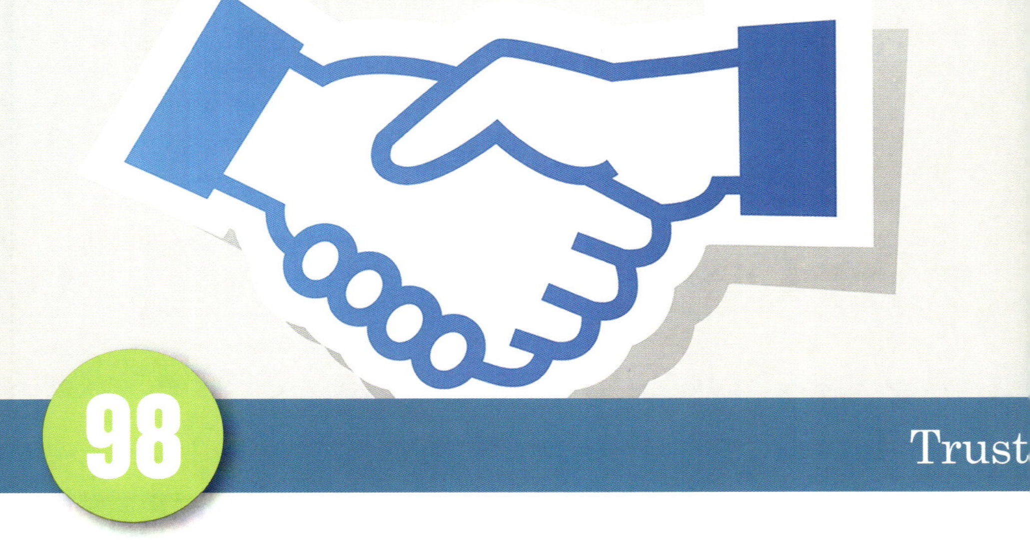

98 Trust

Lack of trust is one of the primary barriers to people accepting treatment plans. They must have high levels of trust in you as a professional and a person. Here are nine ways to be more trustworthy:

1. Under-promise and over-deliver. Trust is created when peoples' experiences exceed their expectations.
2. Tell the truth. Don't shade or stretch the truth. It will come back to haunt you.
3. Listen first. People don't care how much you know until they know how much you care.
4. Clarify expectations. In advance, show and tell people what the road ahead looks like.
5. Don't be pushy. This is the primary way dental professionals lower the trust factor with patients. Don't push. Be confident. Be assertive. Tell them what you believe. Above all, treat them the way you would want to be treated.
6. Keep commitments. Being on time is an example. Or apologize if you're not on time.
7. Offer guarantees. If you guarantee certain types of treatment, tell your patients. Or better yet, give them a written guarantee.
8. Demonstrate stability. If appropriate, communicate to people how long you have practiced dentistry in the area.
9. Dress professionally.
    - Wear comfortable dress shoes, slacks and a dress shirt when doing patient examinations. Then put on the disposable gown when doing clinical dentistry. If a tie fits your practice brand, wear one.
    - Front office people should wear business clothing suitable for the patients you see.
    - DA's and Hygienists can wear professional looking scrubs with your office logo.

Enhancing your trust level is vitally important if you want to do more comprehensive cases. Remember: the bigger the case, the more trust you need to generate.

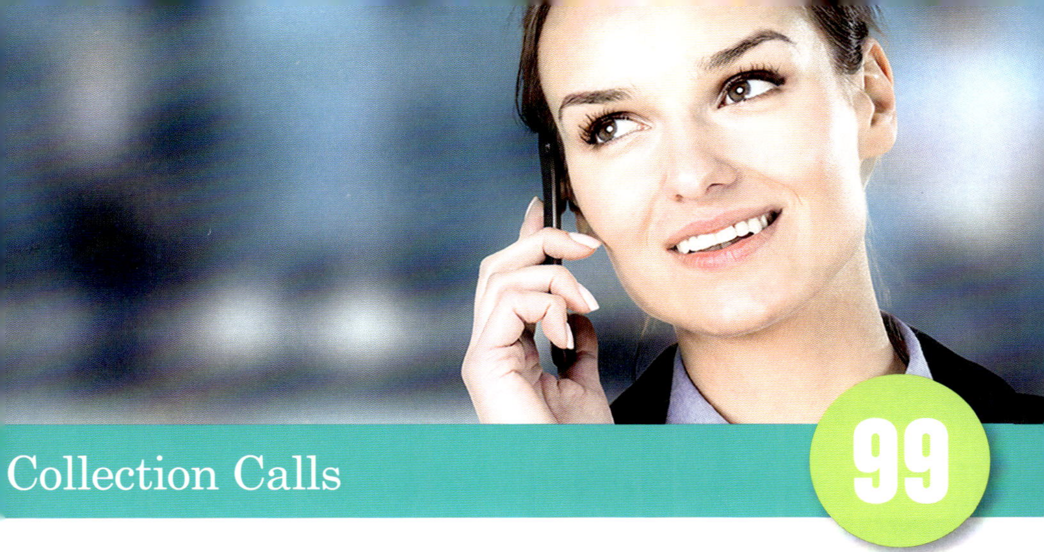

Collection Calls

99

Hopefully, you collect payment for services before or on the day of service, so your office isn't financing patients' dental care. Or you may have a third party handle billing and collections.

If you do have to make collection calls from your office, here is the process to do it well:

Team Member: "Hello, Mrs. Finneran. This is Eileen from Dr. Harris's office. I'm calling about the balance on your account."

Patient: "I didn't know I had a balance."

Team Member: "Let me explain how the balance happened. After your last visit, the insurance company paid $85 of the $145 total fee. That leaves a balance of $60 on your account. I want to help you clear this up. For your convenience, we accept debit or credit cards over the phone."

Patient: "I can't pay you right now. My cards are maxed out."

Team Member: "I understand. So your account with us doesn't become a problem for you, let's set up a new financial agreement that's comfortable for you."

Patient: "I get paid this Thursday. I'll drop a $30 check this Friday and another one next Friday."

Team Member: Thank you, Mrs. Finneran. Let me review our agreement so we both have the same understanding. We can expect to receive a $30 check this Friday and another one next Friday. This will clear your account with us. Are you comfortable with that agreement?"

Patient: "That will be fine."

Team Member: "I will make a note of the conversation in our system. I appreciate you clearing this up."

Conversation Comments:

- Timely follow-up is important. The longer a past due bill is active, the less chance it will be paid.
- Think of a collection call as an opportunity to clear up a misunderstanding and to offer help.
- When you first speak to the patient, identify yourself and the reason for the call. Then, be silent and let the patient respond.
- Make sure a firm agreement is made before the conversation ends.
- Summarize the agreement and document it in your practice management system.
- Use a calendar or tickler system to make sure the patient follows through.
- Always maintain rapport and be positive.

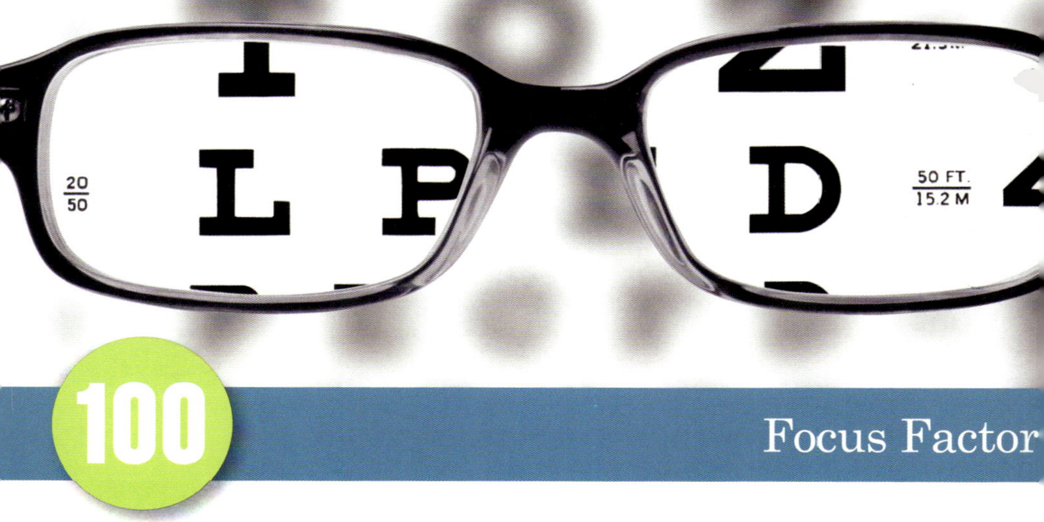

100 Focus Factor

When reinventing your dental practice it helps if you break down what you want to achieve. Trying to do too much all at once risks early burnout.

Focus means exactly that: whittling down your top goals into a single mission. Very often this way of thinking reduces stress, clears the mind, and prepares you for the tasks at hand.

That doesn't mean you should forgo your other goals. It just means you need to value your priorities.

And when you try to do too much, very often it's the most challenging tasks that get overlooked first. It's human nature. We tend to put off what's the most difficult to achieve – especially if that task is included in a laundry list of must-dos.

Put that list on the side (for a moment) and make your first task the only task. That will ensure it gets done.

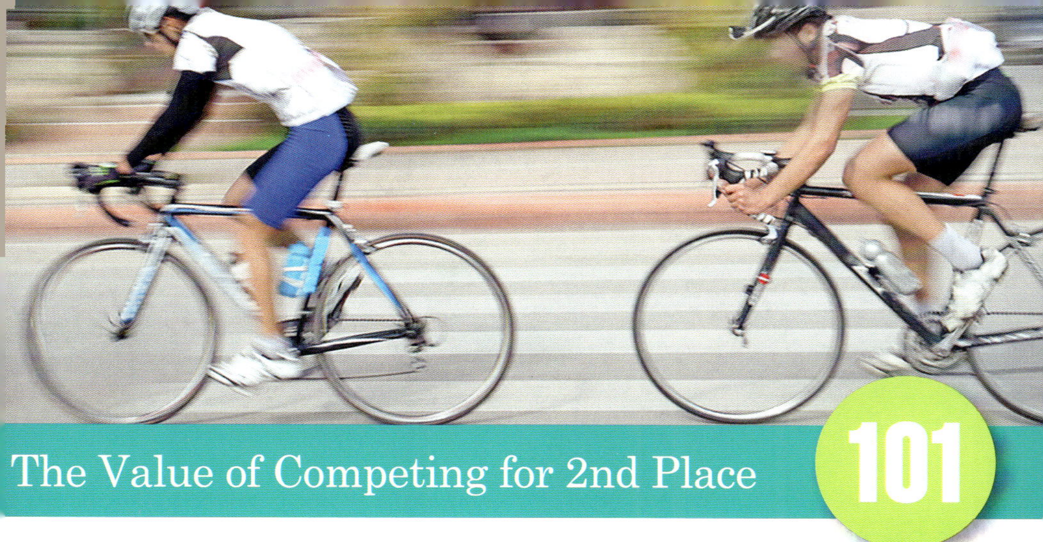

The Value of Competing for 2nd Place 101

At first glance the title of this tip might seem counterintuitive. Who wants to be in second place?

That is, except for the person in third place.

Rank orderings are common in life. In families. In sports. And in the office. Some colleagues work faster and more efficient than others. There's a pecking order.

Aspiring for second place means you've already "beat" out much of the competition.

The key is to find someone in your office who you think works a little harder than you, a little better than you, and aspire to meet or beat their efforts.

As a dental practice manager, it's important to evaluate your staff along these lines. Try to encourage inter-office relationships and chemistry that help employees recognize and understand these connections.

You can even try a more direct approach and organize a meeting that speaks to these needs. Whichever solution you choose, remember the value of competing for second place.

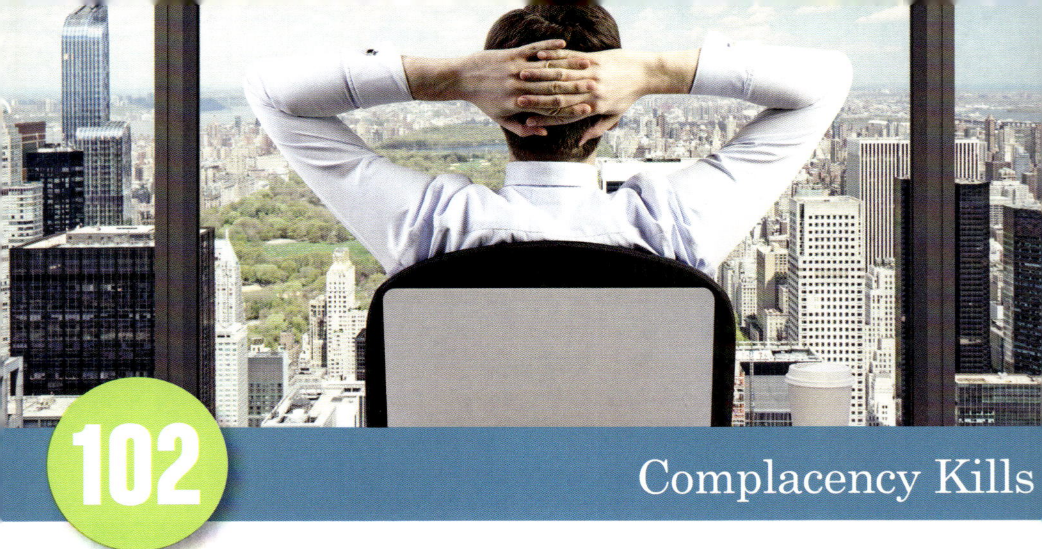

102 Complacency Kills

Congratulations! Your dental practice is doing great. Patient volume is up. New procedures are receiving positive feedback. Patients love the new hygienist, and your front office staff is repeatedly praised for a job well done.

Now what?

While it could be easy to rest on your success and bask in the glory of your business acumen, this is exactly the time when competitors are looking to pounce.

People like to say "it's lonely at the top." But that's only true if your business is innovative enough to *remain on top.*

This is the moment your dental practice needs a gut check moment. What else could you be doing to be even better?

Answering this question requires a bit of research. Take the time to investigate what your competitors are currently doing. Reach out to out-of-market colleagues who may be plugged in to global trends. And most importantly, ask your most loyal patients either in person or through surveys what else they would like to see your dental practice offer. And ideally, how fast would they like to see these improvements implemented.

Complacency kills – especially when you're already on top!

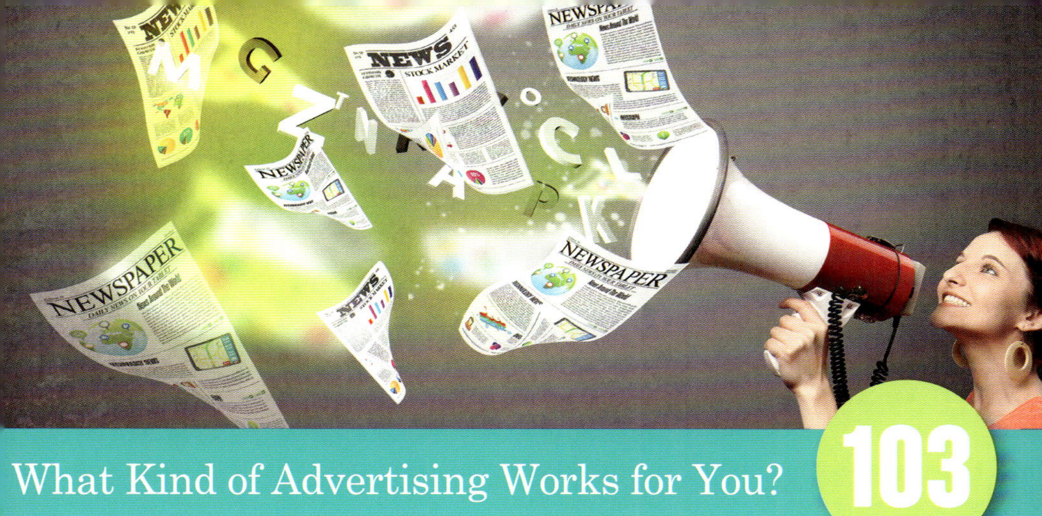

What Kind of Advertising Works for You? 103

Since the advent of radio and television, the degree to which Americans are bombarded with advertising has increased by a staggering figure.

According to one frequently referenced study, the amount of ad exposure has increased from about 500 a day in the 1970s to more than 5,000 a day in 2006, a 90 percent increase. Today, digital marketers estimate that number as high as 10,000 a day.

With this level of information overload it can be easy to become overwhelmed. Picking the right advertising strategy – and in the right channels – is essential for the success of any business.

Dental offices are no exception.

Of course, online advertising garners the most attention. From our phones and tablets, to our laptops and smartwatches, our eyes are never far from a glowing screen. In this medium, banner ads (the advertisement that scrolls across the top or side of a screen) are particularly common and are a pay-per-click endeavor – the ad value increases the more consumers click on the ad.

A newer form of online advertising is called "native advertising." Native advertising blurs the line between original content specific to a website and an advertorial. Native ads are designed to look "native" to the page at hand and be less intrusive to the viewer, hence its name.

But for all the hype that online advertising generates, it's important not to dismiss the tried and true basics of television and radio. A well-timed radio or TV ad, especially in a local market, can be just as effective –or more so— in attracting, retaining and engaging new patients.

Keep this advertising advice in mind as you take your dental practice to new and incredible heights!

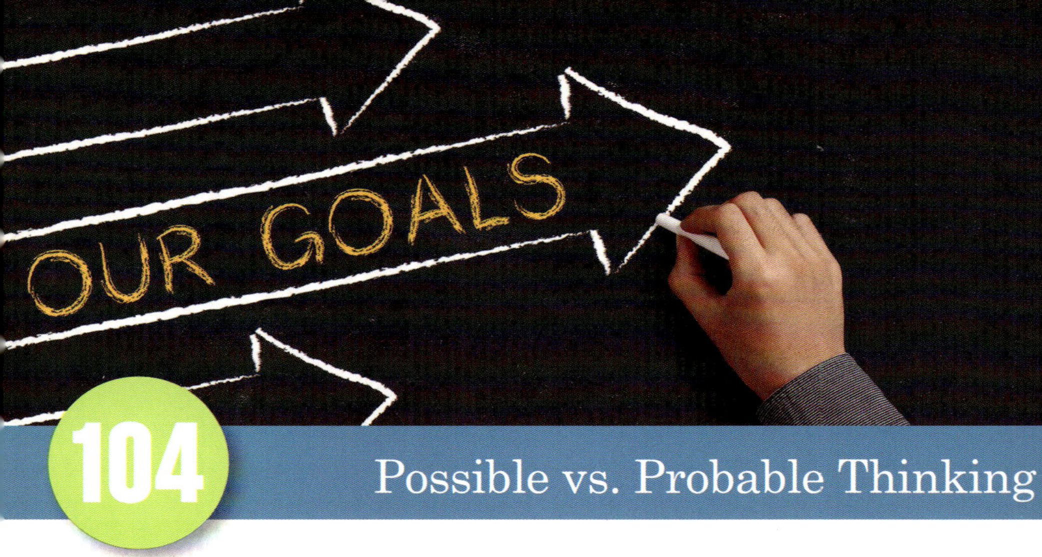

104 Possible vs. Probable Thinking

It's an important psychological distinction, possible vs. probable thinking. Possible thinking is laced with skepticism. In healthy doses, though, it's likely beneficial to your cause, whatever that may be.

But when it comes to not just successful dental practice management, but truly exceptional dentistry, you need a little more. You need probable thinking. And just as important, you need to inspire your staff to think along similar lines.

This isn't a trivial tip. The clichéd "power of positive thinking" has been well studied. Thinking positively (and by extension believing in that positivity) actually moves the needle of performance. It's truly incredible.

What does probable thinking look like?

Probable thinking is about setting goals that at first glance, might feel too grand. But enacting concrete steps in order to realize them actually helps meet the goal. It's similar to how important lists can be for achieving goals. The sense of accomplishment is palpable. Compulsive list makers even tell me that they feel a tingling down the spine and a quickening of the heart, when they check off an important task.

Organize your dental practice along similar lines.

Encourage your staff to write personal daily lists of what they hope to accomplish. Review those lists and offer suggestions on how to achieve those goals. It could be simple goals like:

- Answer all front office phone calls within two rings and be friendlier and more genuine than ever
- Recruit 2 new patients per week
- Follow up on 3 delinquent payments per day and complete at least one of those outstanding bills, or confirm a timeline for completion
- Remove all periodicals older than three months and update accordingly
- Improve office curbside appeal, picking up trash, improving signage, re-painting parking spot lines, etc., etc.

Once you've helped indoctrinate a sense of communal accomplishment, of team spirit, it's likely you will have begun to move your staff from believing in what's possible to what's probable.

Empower your dental practice with the belief that (at least in the near term and foreseeable future) your continued success is CERTAIN!

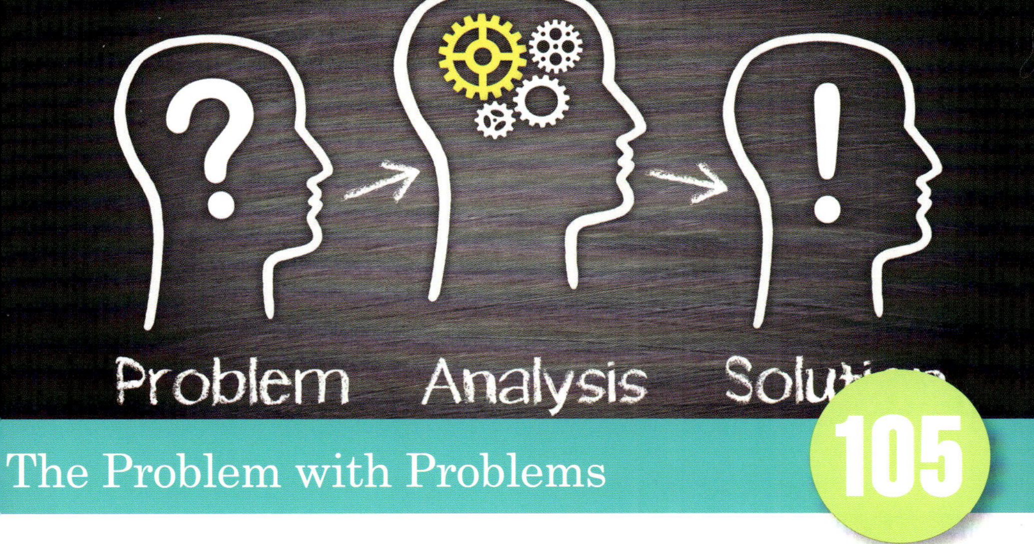

105

The Problem with Problems

"No one understands my business."

"My challenges are unique."

"Nothing like this has every happened before."

Stay in business long enough and chances are you or someone you know will offer pronouncements like this.

Whether we realize it or not, these are defensive statements. They're designed to deflect personal responsibility. The implied logic: our problems are so unique, that they are unsolvable. And since they're unsolvable, it's not our fault that they haven't been solved.

It's bulletproof logic. Until you remind yourself that nine times out of 10, pronouncements like these are rationalizations.

In fact, nearly all problems – in life and in business – are not unique. They've been encountered thousands of times by millions of businesses spread out over the ages.

Problem solving begins with a reality check and a dose of humility. Don't look for complicated solutions when your problems really aren't that complex.

That's not to say your dental practice is a dime a dozen. With the proper management it can become unique. But your problems....

Chances are they're yesterday's news. Get over it.

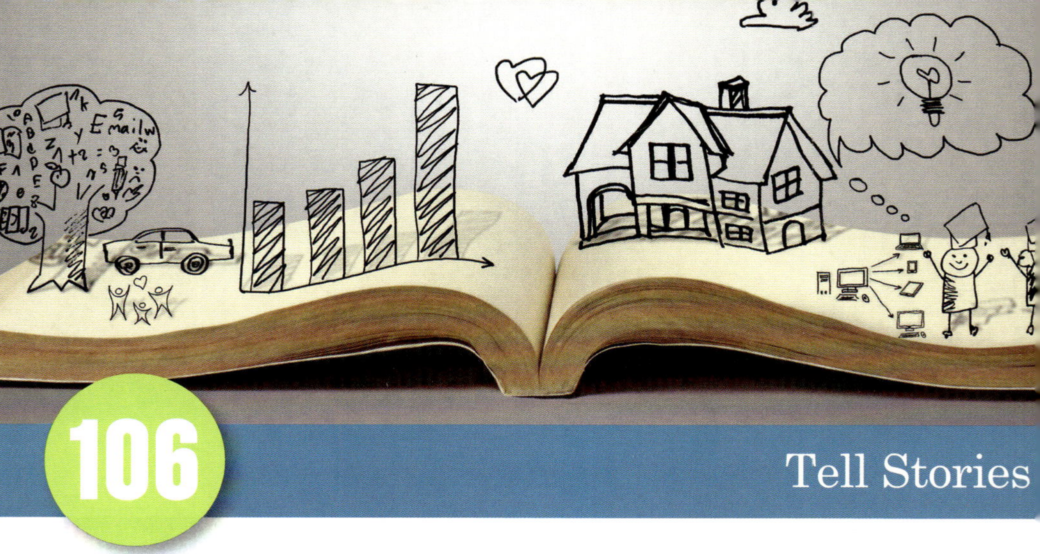

106 Tell Stories

Storytelling is among the most ancient forms of communication. If a picture is worth a thousand words, then a story is worth a thousand pictures. When it comes to case acceptance, stories that highlight the same situation as your current patient can make all the difference.

The Positive Story

Here's an example: "Maria, we had a woman named Roxana in our office two years ago who had loose dentures like you. Roxana couldn't eat what she wanted and was in constant fear of her dentures coming out. Roxana even stopped wearing them unless she had to. She heard about implant-retained dentures, but was afraid to take the first step. Finally, Roxana came to see us. We placed two implants on top and two on the bottom. She wore her old dentures while the implants became attached to the bone. Then we made her new upper and lower snap-in dentures. Now Roxana loves how they look, feel and work. She can eat what she wants and never worries about their stability. Maria, I know this is a big step. When you get your new snap-in dentures, I'm sure you will feel like Roxana, too".

There are four steps to the above story:

1. There was a patient of ours who was in the same situation as you.
2. She took the action I want you to take.
3. She received several benefits from taking the action.
4. When you take the same action, you will receive the same benefits.

The Negative Story

You can also use negative stories to influence hesitant patients to take action. There are four steps to the negative story:

1. There was a patient of ours who was in the same situation as you.
2. She didn't take the action I want you to take.
3. Several negative consequences resulted in her decision.
4. Don't let the same negative consequences happen to you.

The art of story telling is one of the most important communication skills you can master. It will help patients improve their health, increase your acceptance rate, and make everyone's in-office time more enjoyable.

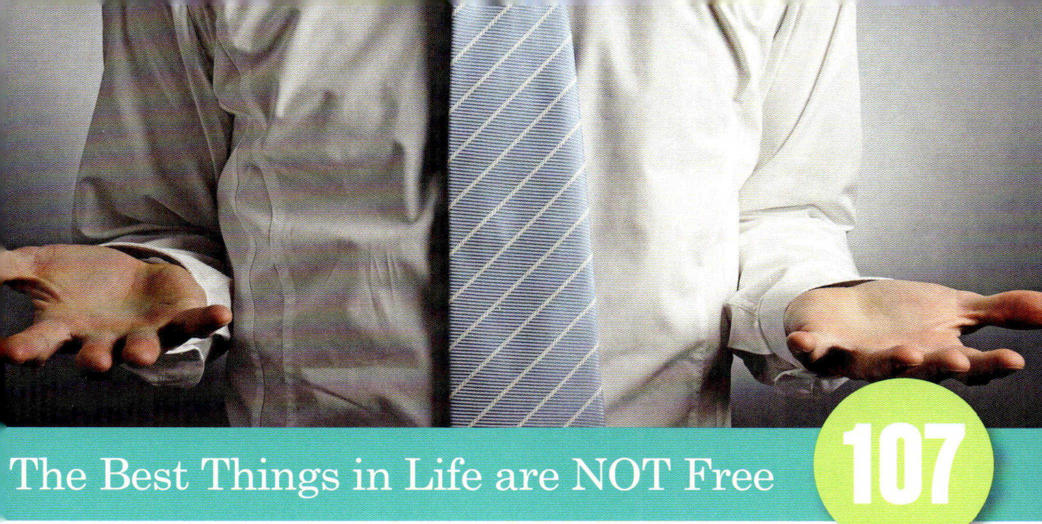

The Best Things in Life are NOT Free

107

This tip title isn't meant to be a downer. Driven by the law of supply and demand, economists will generally agree with its sentiment.

The best things in life are NOT free. Especially when it comes to business advice.

Of course, platitudes are easy to come by. And to the extent that they help inspire a frame of mind, they can be useful. Ben Franklin is the American original when it comes to providing such advice.

Concrete action steps are harder to come by. Often it requires spending money and doing your homework. After all, if everyone were receiving such stellar counsel, then we'd all be successful, right?

When building your dental practice, don't be afraid to say, "I don't know." And don't be afraid to seek out professional assistance when making critical decisions.

Outside help might require more time and money. But as Ben Franklin might say, "an investment in knowledge pays the best interest."

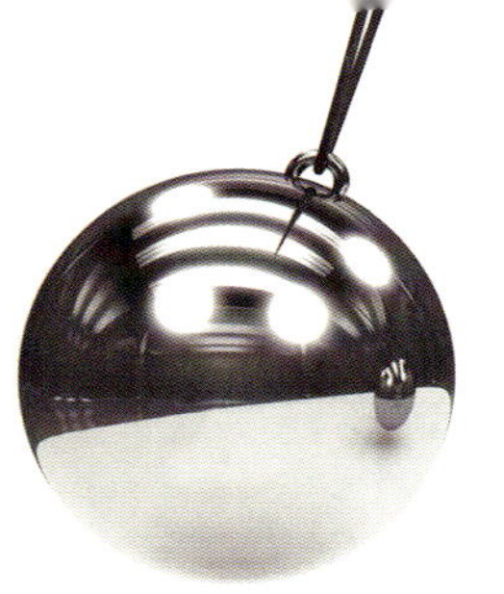
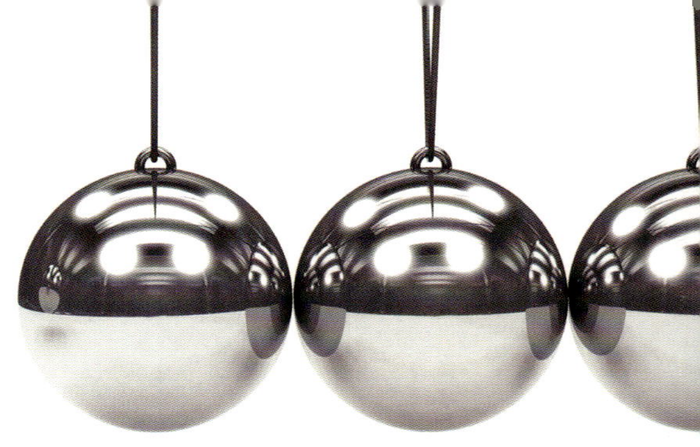

108 First-rate Insights from Newton's Third Law

It's a ten-word sentence we all learned in high school physics: "for every action, there is an equal and opposite reaction."

Newton's third law of gravity distilled into its simplest form.

But there's a dental practice management lesson here too.

As business owners and doctors, there are many things in life we don't have control over. If the economy goes belly up, there's little we can do. If a patient has a last-minute cancellation, we'll be hard pressed to find a replacement. If neighborhood demographics change, your practice could struggle maintaining its patient base.

How we react to situations largely out of our control is just as important as the situation itself.

So while we can't control the economy at large, we can take steps to mitigate emerging challenges. (That could mean reducing overhead, closing a secondary practice, or even letting some people go or cutting back on hours.) If the demographics of your neighborhood are changing, stay a step ahead of those changes and begin altering your practice makeup to better reflect the patients you treat.

Don't worry about what you can't control. Focus instead on how you react to those situations.

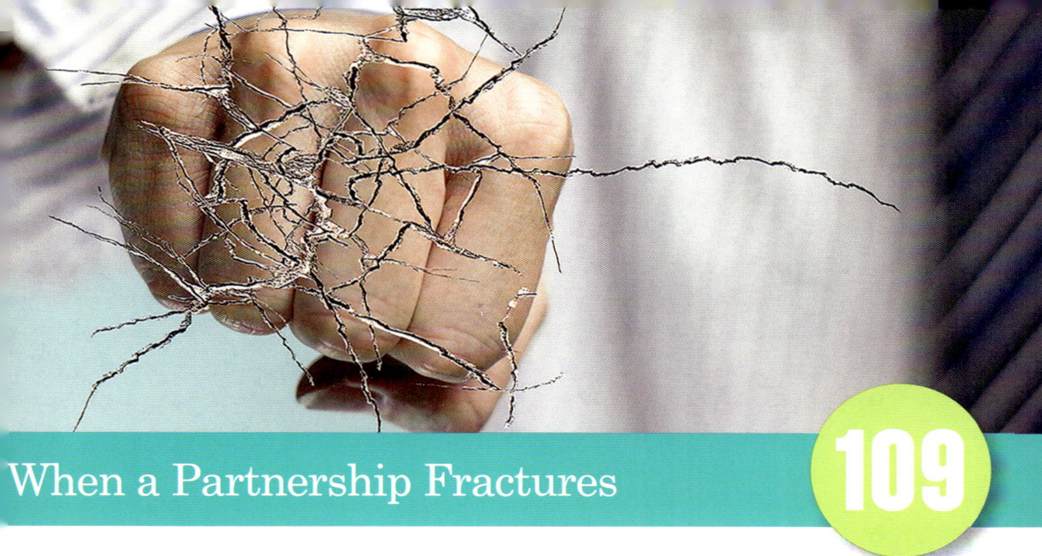

When a Partnership Fractures

109

Unfortunately, teeth aren't the only things that can fracture in a dental office. Business partnerships can go south too and it's a very unfortunate event.

Sometimes you don't even realize it's happening. Slowly, little by little, the dynamic between two people, once amicable, changes. Miscommunication or non-communication develops. Suspicion is bread. Defense mechanisms kick in. And before long, your practice is on the skids.

Confronting an issue like this isn't easy. In fact, it's one of the hardest for any business owner to handle.

At these moments, it's important not to sabotage an already tenuous situation by making it worse.

Take a step back and be the bigger person. Openly engage your business partner and request a meeting. Keep the conversation civil and use your best judgment. Ultimately you might conclude that salvaging the partnership is impossible. In those situations make sure you have all the proper documentation in place to protect your own interests.

Don't think you can do this alone. Seek legal counsel to review all paperwork to ensure your business rights are protected.

Most important is to not let a bad situation fester. Confront it. Own up to it. And take steps to ensure your patients don't get caught in the middle of something that can look and a feel a lot like a marriage breakup. "He said, she said," spats is not the way to maintain quality care.

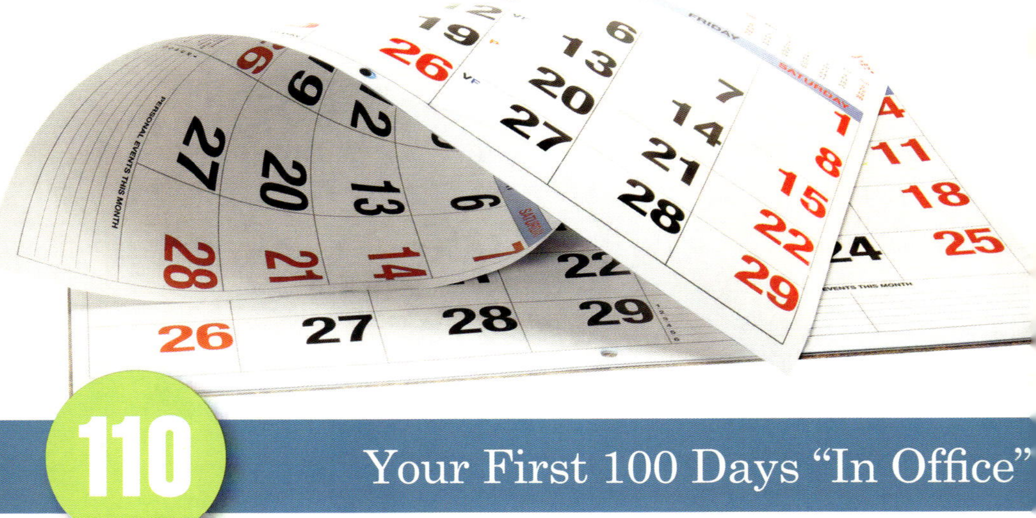

110 Your First 100 Days "In Office"

As this book's printing is coming in the midst of one of the most exciting (and incredulous) election cycles in generations, this tip addresses your first 100 days in office as dental practice manager.

The first 100 days is a term that comes from President Franklin Roosevelt and his efforts to pass numerous pieces of critical legislation during his first 100 days in office. Thanks to that swift action, today all presidents' first 100 days are reviewed with scrutiny. Arguably it's when a newly elected president's power and influence are at their greatest – both in terms of persuading the American people, and congress.

So what will your first 100 days in office look like?

If you're taking over an existing practice, knowing your practice's financials will be critical. Next will be carefully assessing overhead, and making sure your staff makeup meets existing patient demand, that your licensing and credentials are up to date, and that your equipment is safe to operate.

Above all, setting the right tone is essential. Remember, you're taking over from someone else. In some cases, there's decades of loyalty built up between current staff and a former owner. Like the president who inherits the ship of state, so too, will you need to introduce yourself to your staff. Earn their trust and respect with a mix of optimism and pragmatism.

Of course, having a successful first 100 days does not guarantee the next 1,000 days or the next 10,950 (the number of days in 30 years) will be perfect. But there's no point in denying the importance of starting off your term in office with the best foot forward!

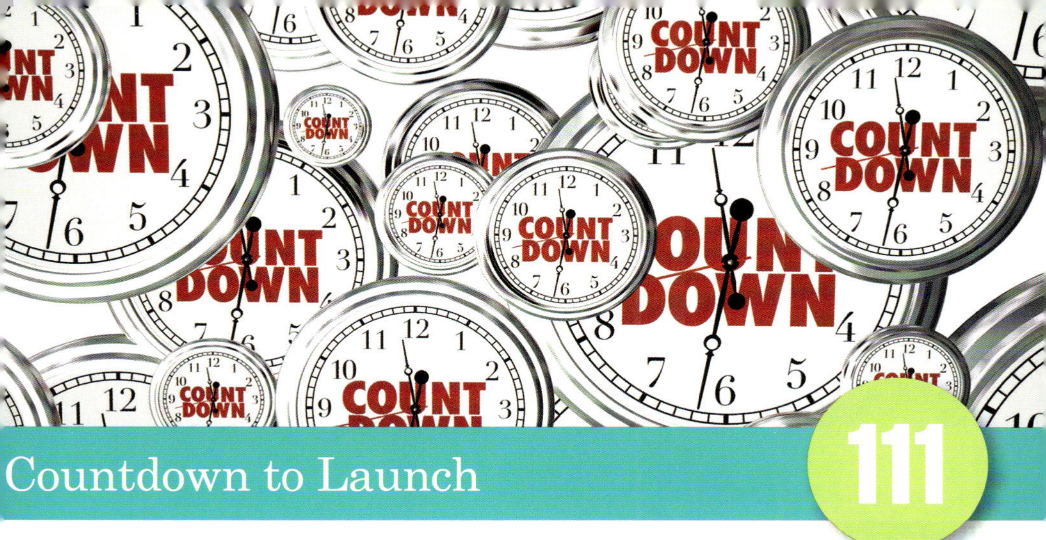

Countdown to Launch

111

The previous tip discussed the importance of the first 100 days. What you will do once in office. But there's a preliminary meeting to have before that. It's what I call the countdown to launch.

Generally launches fall under the "hard launch" or "soft launch" categories.

The "soft launch" is filled with unbridled and perhaps over-the-top optimism. This is where no one can do any wrong. It's where all ideas are given serious consideration – even if those ideas are unrealistic.

The downside of such a meeting rests with its amateur nature. If your dental practice launch has reached the countdown phase, chances are you're beyond this type of meeting.

A better approach is the "hard launch." As the name implies, this is where the hard questions get asked. And better still, answered. The hard launch is the dress rehearsal for the 100 days that's to come. Or, if you prefer another analogy, think about NASA's "countdown" to launch. Every countdown includes a carefully proscribed dialogue, a precise checklist of what needs to be done, and the order in which these things needs to happen to ensure the safety of the flight crew and for that matter, all personnel involved.

Your dental practice isn't planning the next manned mission to Mars. But for you, your patients, and your staff, your dental practice is a universe onto itself. A place where patient's dreams are realized and employees are (ideally) inspired to show up to work.

Shoot for the stars when it comes to your dental practice success and be sure to ask the hard questions in a pre-launch countdown.

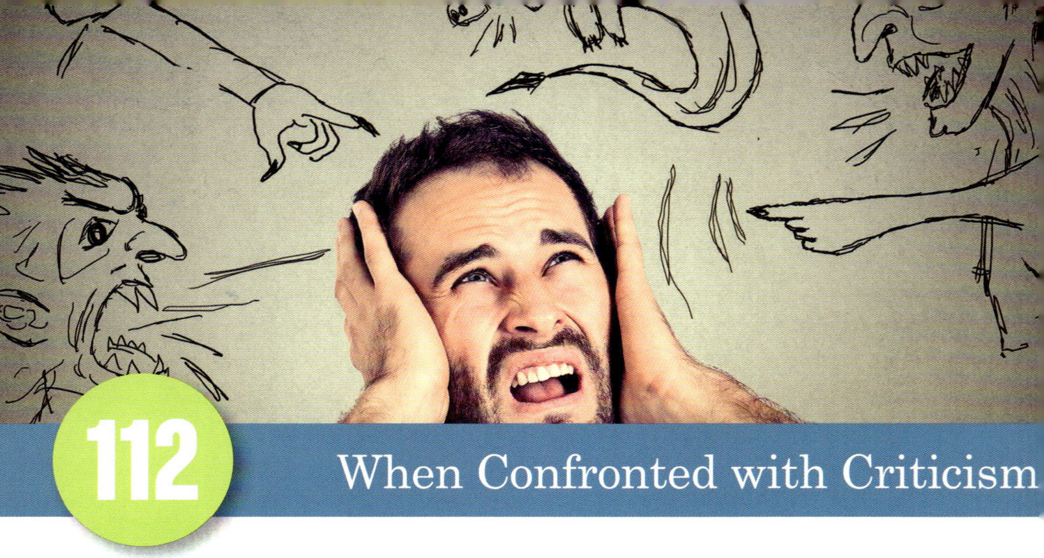

112 When Confronted with Criticism

It's not something most people enjoy. But eventually, everyone, everywhere, gets criticized. More often than not that criticism comes unsolicited.

As dental practice managers, our businesses deal with many moving parts, straddling patient care, business growth, and technological investment. Therefore from lab technicians, to your front office staff, to patients, and your hygienists, criticism can come from many different directions. It can feel like a whirlwind.

How you respond to criticism is critically important. First, you have to judge the validity of the source. Do you trust this person's judgment? If not, then their criticism has less merit. (It also begs the question why such a person is on your team.) But if you do value what's been said, take their observations to heart.

Doing so encourages humility, opens your mind to new perspectives, and allows you to assess how you could improve, or what you could have done differently.

The worst thing you can do is to become defensive or argumentative. Criticism is not a forum inviting debate. Or at least it shouldn't be. Strike a tone of genuine interest in addressing your shortcomings. Be appreciative of the advice and take proactive steps to make those corrections.

A humble boss who admits they're not perfect and is willing to change can be a huge benefit to your dental practice success.

Criticism can be the catalyst for change. Embrace it!

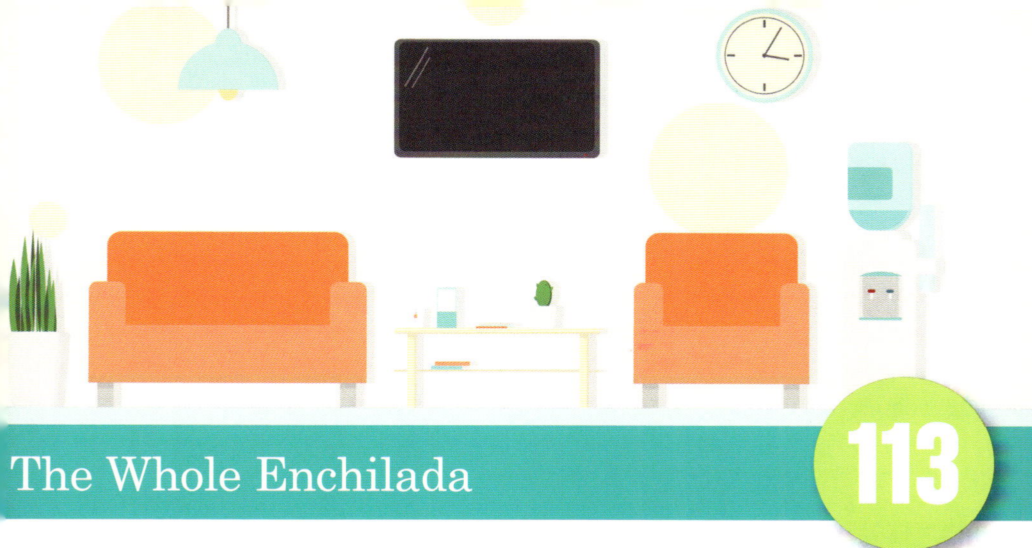

The Whole Enchilada

113

Here's an expression that needs a rethink: "finishing touches."

The phrase implies an afterthought. But here's the truth: a finishing touch can be the difference between a sale and an interested patient who says, "Maybe next time."

Finishing touches should be "first touches."

Realtors know this well. Studies show that on average, a home with excellent landscaping will bring in 5 percent more in value and 7 percent more value compared to a home whose landscaping needs serious work.

If your dental practice is in a large office building you probably won't have much control over the actual landscaping. But "corporate landscaping" can include suggestions like:

- Trees/plants (fake or real) outside your office door
- New carpets, new magazines, new furniture
- Flat screen TVs, with a mix of cable television programming and informational videos
- Pleasant background/white noise sounds
- Complimentary bottled water
- Free Wi-Fi

Transform your finishing touches into first touches and these little improvements might go a long way toward enhancing your dental practice curbside appeal.

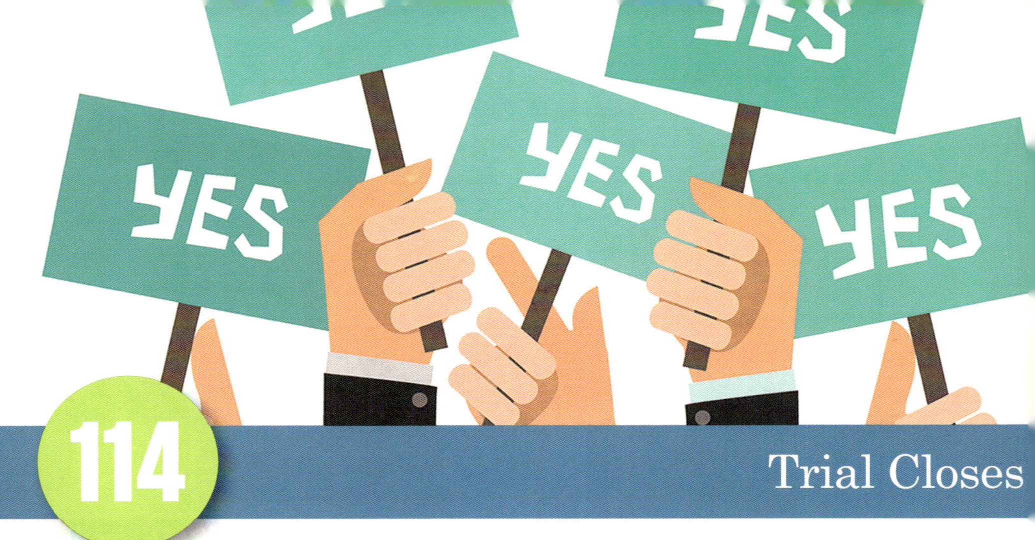

114 Trial Closes

Trial Closes are questions that help patients make small steps toward case acceptance. This is way more effective than asking patients to make a huge leap. Trial Closes discover the mood, hesitations and level of interest in the treatment plan you're presenting.

Examples of Trial Closes are:

- "Are you with me so far?"
- "Have I answered all your questions?"
- "How does that sound?"
- "Do you see what I mean?"
- "Does that make sense?"
- "What haven't I covered yet that is important to you?"
- When you give a benefit such as, "You're implant-retained dentures will snap into place." Ask, "How will that benefit you?"
- "If we can fit this care into your budget, is this what you'd like to do?"

If you ask a Trial Close Question that has a "Yes" or "No" answer, make sure the answer will probably be "Yes." Several small "yes's" early in your case conversations will often lead to a big "yes" at the end.

After you ask a Trial Close Question, be quiet. Let them have a moment to think about it and respond. It's ideal to ask three or four trial closes before you ask a Final Close Question. We will discuss Final Closes in the next tip.

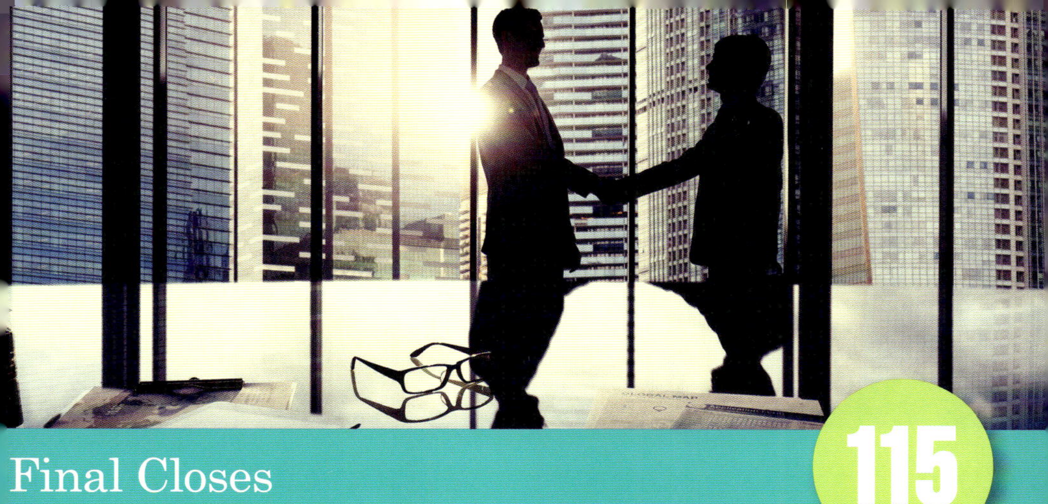

Final Closes

115

After you have asked a series of Trial Close questions, and you feel the patient is ready to accept treatment, ask a Final Close Question. Examples are:

Alternative Choice Close

1. "Which (payment) option works best for you?"
2. "Would you like to start with the veneers or implants first?"
3. "Would you like to complete your dental care all at once, or would phasing the care be better for you?"

Trade-Off Close

1. If the patient asks for a discount, ask, "If we can give you the 10% discount, can you start treatment today?"
2. If the patient says, "We're leaving the country next month." Ask, "If we can start tomorrow and be done in two weeks, will that work for you?"
3. Dental Care Agreement Close – As you explain the treatment plan, use a printed Dental Care Agreement as visual reinforcement. Fill out the Dental Care Agreement. Then say, "Mrs. Garcia, just OK the paperwork right here."
4. Special Event in the Future Close – If they have a special event in the future, ask, "If we start today, we can get those veneers done in time for the wedding. OK?"
5. Something for Nothing Close – "If I can get you the whitening for free, will you agree to the treatment plan?"

After you ask a Final Close Question, be quiet. Let them have a moment to think about it and respond. If you have to respond to an objection, ask another Final Close Question. Don't let the conversation fizzle out.

When asking questions, always come from the right place in your heart. Care about your patients. Help them make decisions that will improve their lives. Don't just make a sale. Make a friend.

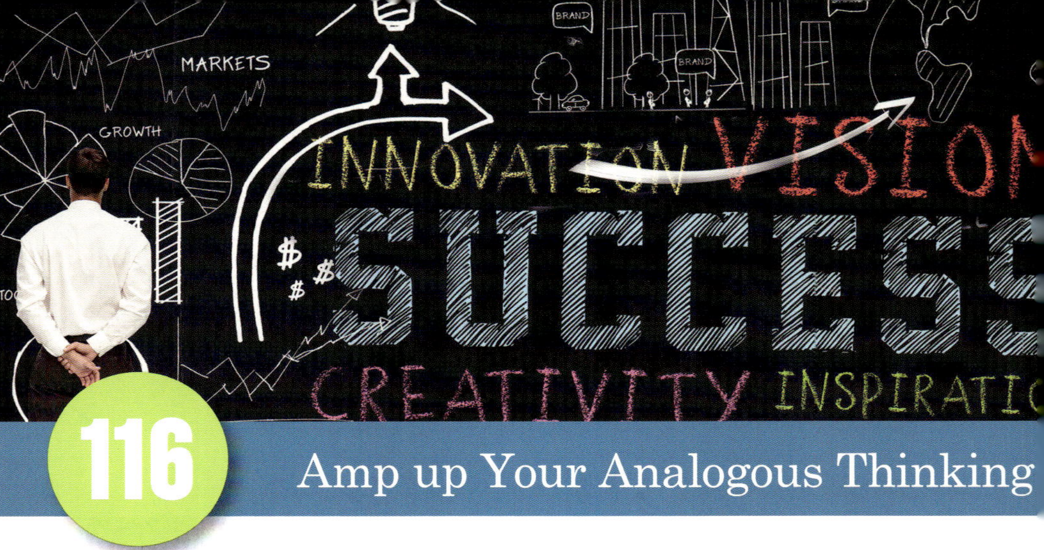

116 Amp up Your Analogous Thinking

In biology, analogous structures are similar biological components that have the same appearance and function. A common example is the wings of insects and birds used for flying. They evolved separately and don't share a common ancestor.

But that doesn't mean a scientist studying insect wings can't learn a thing or two by studying bird wings.

Business leaders have long applied this thinking to humans. Analogous industries are those that share a deep similarity but at the surface have little in common. Repeatedly it is shown that when you bring people within these industries together innovation skyrockets.

Examples of this innovation at work are numerous:

- The cushioning of a Reebok basketball shoe was inspired by intravenous fluid bags
- Semiconductor firm Qualcomm's color display technology is based in part on the Morpho butterfly's wings
- A leak-proof water bottle borrows technology from a shampoo bottle top

So whether you call it analogous thinking or "peripheral knowledge," it never hurts to discuss your dental practice challenges with innovative people who seemingly have little professionally in common with you and your business.

It also helps if you personally cultivate your own knowledge base about topics that might not relate to dentistry per se, but they interest you all the same.

When you least expect it, an innovative solution to a vexing problem might be just around the corner!

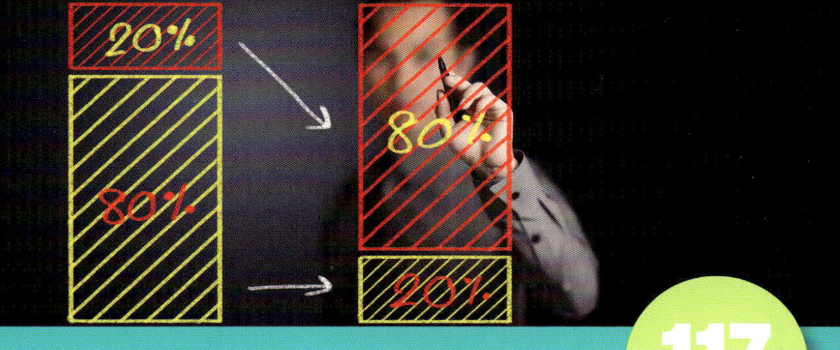

The 80-20 Rule Applied to Dentistry

If you're new to dental practice management and the business world in general, you may not have heard of the 80-20 rule.

Also known as the "Pareto principle," or the "law of the vital few," the principle states that in any situation, 80 percent of outcomes are attributed to 20 percent of the causes of an event. In business this means that roughly 80 percent of your revenue comes from 20 percent of your customers.

While dental offices provide a very specific service to the community, it's likely a breakdown of your annual revenue would show a similar trend.

Think about it.

Some of your patients are needier, have more money to spend, and value the aesthetic/cosmetic importance of a healthy mouth and radiant smile. Other patients come in twice a year for their cleanings, demonstrate good at-home care, and don't require much more than a "tune-up" in your office. These patients might spend less than $300 a year whereas the first group might spend $3,000 or more.

Does this mean dentists should forget about their "less valuable" patients? Of course not. But the 80-20 rule, if it applies to your dental practice, is something to consider when designing a solid marketing message. This is where it helps to have a deep, highly granular understanding of your patients.

Understanding your patients' needs, goals, and long-term desires doesn't require sophisticated software or even the latest customer relationship management system. (It can help) All it requires is a superior, caring staff – men and women who take the time to get to know their patients well and diligently record these observations.

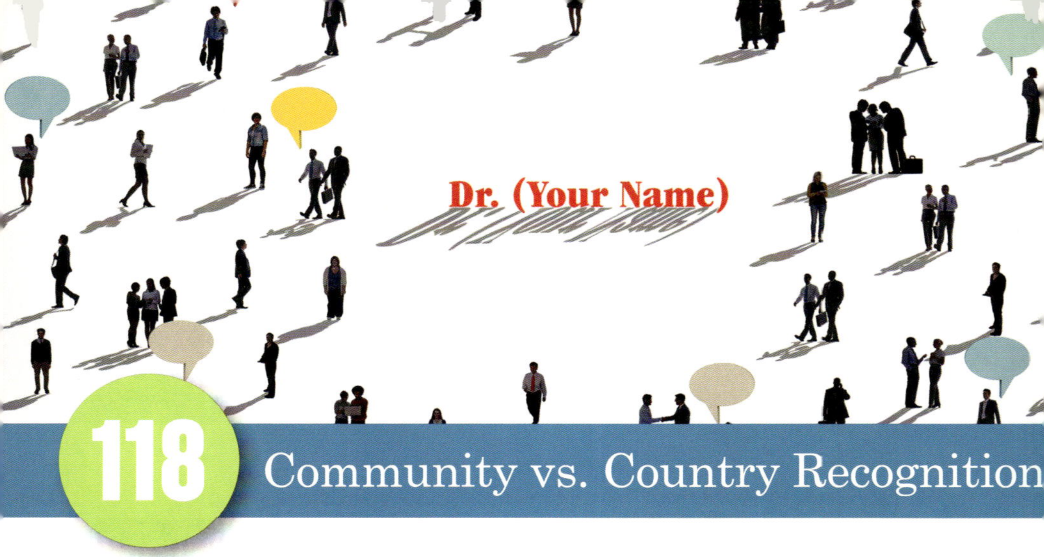

118 Community vs. Country Recognition

In the age of instant digital communication, it's easy to become enamored by the idea that your voice, your actions, your thoughts, can be beamed around the world and accessible by anybody on a myriad of devices.

Today, the number of Facebook friends, and Snapchat and Twitter followers one has is worn like a badge of achievement.

But for all the power the web has to promote Brand You, it's important to remember lowercase brand you.

What do I mean?

I mean that to be a superstar dental practice, you don't need to focus on reaching millions of Americans from California to Maine. Only several hundred patients in your local area. Don't lose site of community recognition. These are the patients that love you. That will support you no matter what, and will continue to refer your services to friends and family for decades to come.

To be sure, the web can and should be a vital resource in achieving this aim.

But there's a host of things a dentist can do – other than practice dentistry – that can help ensure that they're locally respected, and considered a pillar of the community.

My advice: get involved!

If you're married with children, consider becoming a key, positive figure in their schooling. Join the school board. Attend planning and zoning board meetings for your town. Perhaps coach or assistant coach a team sport. Participate in anti-drug campaigns, and organize the annual beach or park cleanup.

Whatever programs you choose, work hard to become a leader in those areas too. Get noticed around town. Here's an easy test: if you're not one of the 10 people that people in your town can rattle off as someone they've at least heard of, you're not doing enough.

Of course, there are only so many hours in a day. And your dental practice and your immediate family take precedence.

Dental practices might well be the last bastion of "old-fashioned" medicine where being "of the community" is as important as being "in the community."

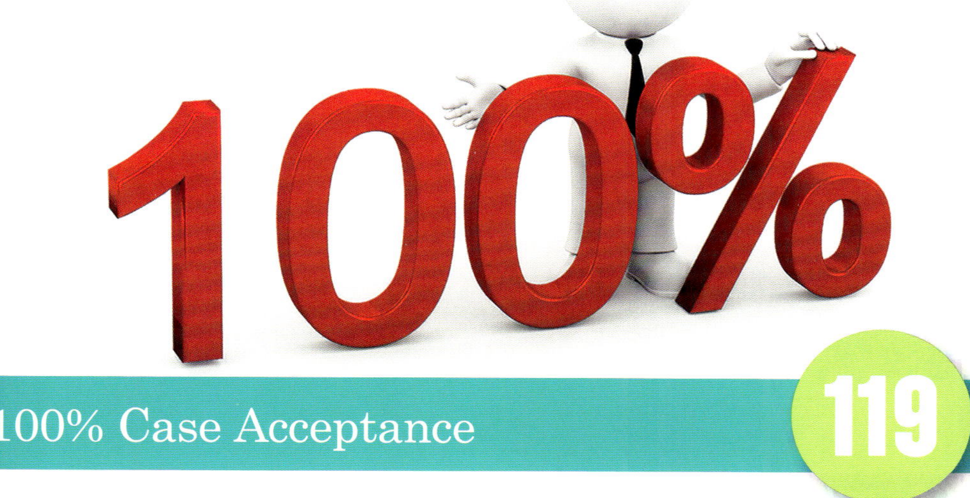

100% Case Acceptance

119

How would you respond if I said that you could achieve 100% case acceptance? You'd think I was nuts, right? There is a way that you can experience 100% case acceptance, but it may involve a change in your definition of success.

To some dentists, failure and success are black and white. They think, "I present comprehensive dentistry to most patients in a very respectful manner. If they accepted all or most of the recommended care, I'm successful. If they don't, I feel like a failure."

Here's another way of viewing this situation. "I have one or more conversations with people depending on the complexity of their cases. In a nutshell, I explain their treatment options and costs; ask respectful questions, listen carefully; and give them what they want. If they don't want to do anything, I'm successful because they stay in our practice and may complete the care in the future."

Options, Options, Options

It's advantageous to start your examination process with, "Is there anything right now that concerns you? I'll make sure I check." After the exam, explain the condition of the patient's mouth to them and give them proof with x-rays and intraoral camera photos.

Tell them that all treatment is elective. Give people requiring comprehensive dentistry five options with the advantages and disadvantages of each:

Option #1 – Do nothing.
Option #2 – Bare minimum dentistry that gets patients out of trouble and stops active disease (decay, abscesses, periodontal problems) from progressing. Large fillings, periodontal therapy, root canals and extractions are examples of Option #2 care.

Option #3 – Higher-end one-tooth-at-a-time dentistry such as crowns and onlays.

Option #4 – Higher-end quadrant dentistry and implants.

Option #5 – Full-mouth reconstruction (possibly with implants) and cosmetic dentistry.

With each option, throw out a ballpark dollar amount and check how they respond verbally and non-verbally. Then ask open-ended questions like, "What are you thinking?" or "What would you like to do?" Finally, work with them to create a treatment plan that fits their desires and finances. There are no right or wrong answers. One hundred percent of the people do what is right for them. In the long run, they will end up doing more dentistry, and you will be much happier."

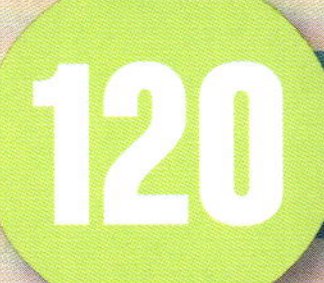

Little Problems of Big Busines

Here's a fact that might surprise you. New York City's Delaware Aqueduct (currently under repair) leaks enough water – about 20 million gallons per day – to supply all the average water usage for cities the size of Albany, New York, Wilmington, North Carolina, Lansing, Michigan, and Cambridge, Massachusetts.

Keeping with the New York theme: the Metropolitan Transit Authority pumps out eight million gallons of groundwater from the city's subway system per day. And this is on a dry day!

Were the MTA pumps to fail or to take a day off, the city's subway system would flood. When the Delaware Aqueduct leak is finally plugged, the city will save 7.3 billion gallons of water.

On first impression, in a city of 8 million, a leaking pipe and a failed water pump might seem like trivial concerns. But as evidenced by the above anecdotes, little setbacks can become very large problems.

It's a lesson that all businesses should learn. Your dental practice is no different.

So while it might not be the most enjoyable way to spend an afternoon or weekend off, take the time to review the little problems in your dental practice; minor snags that in terms of day-to-day operation really don't amount to much. Actually, the more minor the problem, the better.

Evaluate the issue. Try to envision what would happen if that problem were to persist year after year, decade after decade – like the Delaware Aqueduct leakage.

Once you've identified the leak – plug it and plug it fast!

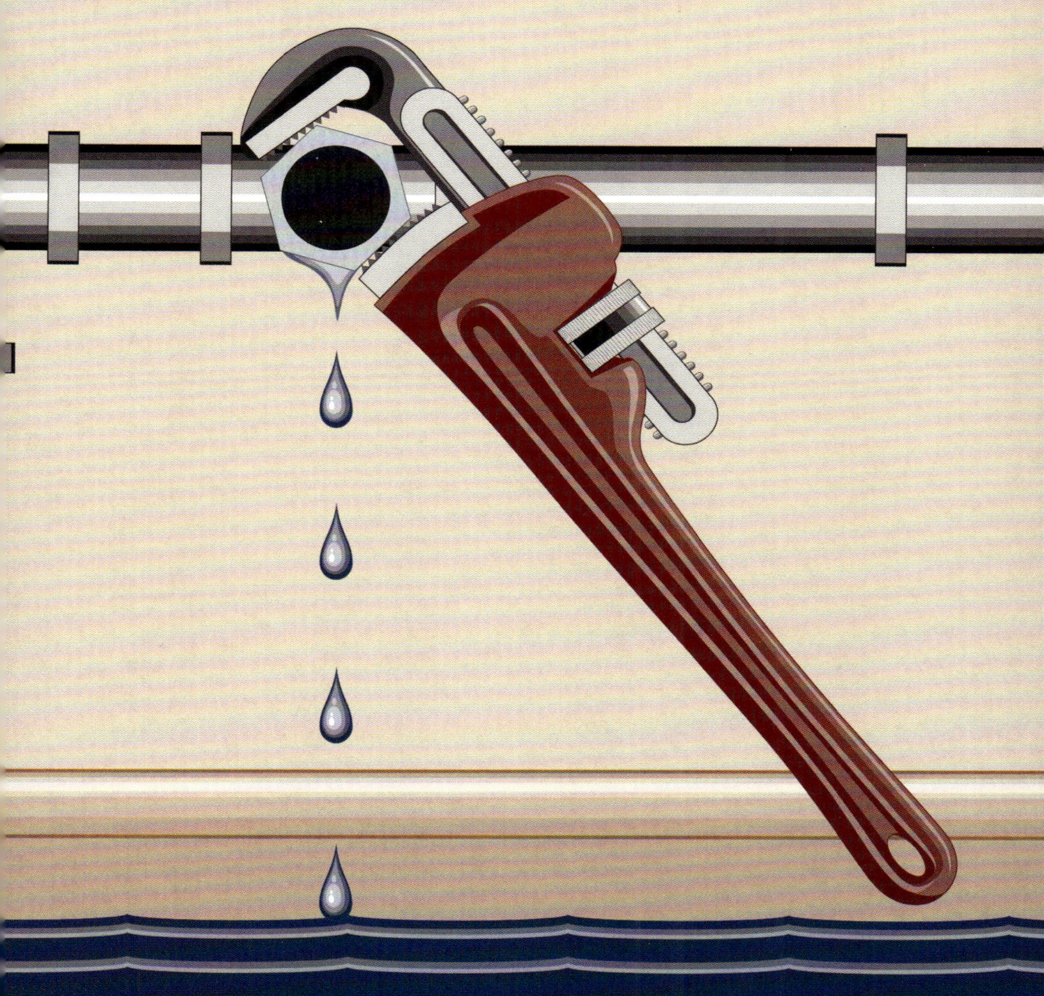

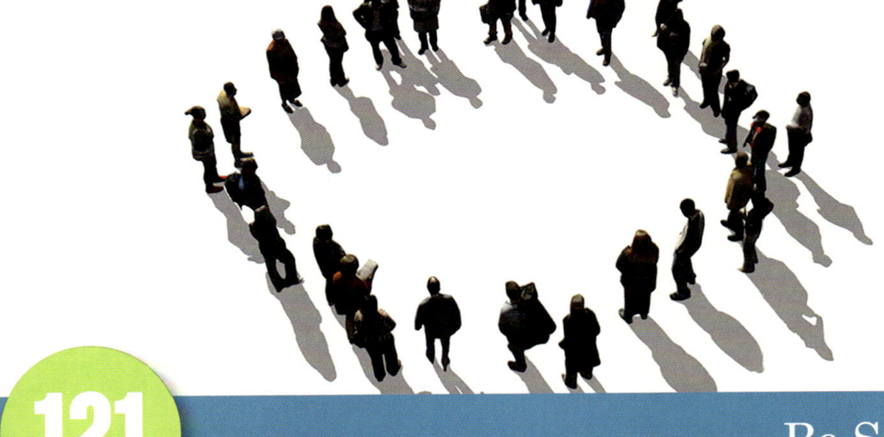

121 Be Smart

We've all heard the stories - tragic tales of dentists who, in their zeal to create practices that only do large cases, severely damage or destroy their traditional practices. These dentists are good people. They believe in their dreams. They're excited about creating those practices glowingly described in the magazines. They work hard. They invest huge sums of money. But they don't know what they're doing. **And people who are just excited but don't know what they're doing are dangerous!**

The basic principle to remember is this: **As you intelligently grow your high-end restorative and implant practice, take excellent care of your traditional practice.**

Imagine a big circle which represents your traditional practice. The patients in this circle have "bread and butter" dentistry in their mouths. You've probably talked to them about comprehensive dentistry, but they didn't have the finances or interest to proceed now. They faithfully come to their re-care visits and have restorations done when something goes wrong.

Now imagine a smaller circle inside the large circle. The patients in this circle have their mouths restored to ideal form and function with your finest implant, restorative and cosmetic dentistry. These are those big cases you love to do.

There are two reasons you want to take great care of your big circle as you grow your small circle:

1. The patients who enter your small circle are going to come from your big circle. If you destroy your big circle, you cut off the supply of new small circle patients.
2. The income you receive from the big circle patients will carry you through the period of time needed to build your high-end restorative practice.

As your small circle gets larger, the area in your traditional practice circle becomes smaller. Now patients come into your small circle from your traditional practice circle and from outside the practice because your reputation is growing.

I hope you see the logic and power of allowing your practice to morph into a high-end implant and restorative practice. When you allow the morphing to naturally occur, you don't have to force the issue. You can also stop the morphing process at any point in time.

The path you take to your dream practice will be unique to you. There is no one ideal path for everybody. There is one best path for you. Be smart as you progress down the path.

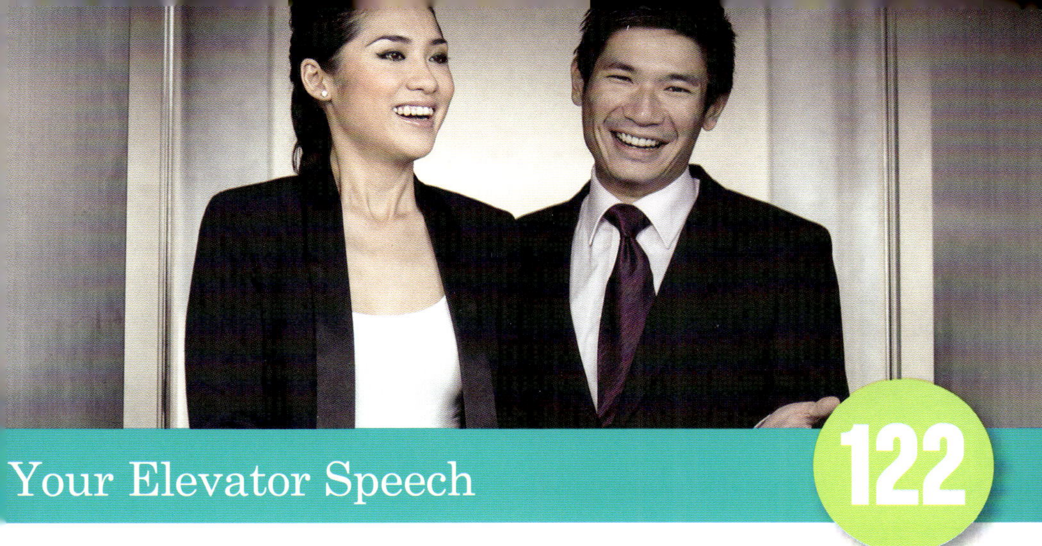

Your Elevator Speech

122

You're on an elevator going from the 23rd floor to the lobby. An extremely friendly co-rider asks, "What do you do?" You only have a few seconds to answer, grab their attention and move the conversation forward. Most dentists would say, "I'm a dentist." That's a quick answer, but it probably won't corral their attention or jump-start the conversation.

Welcome to the wonderful world of the Elevator Speech. You might be thinking, "Sounds great, but this never happens to me." Well, maybe not in an elevator, but I'll bet it's happened in other situations like:

- at a group meeting
- when you make a new friend
- when you talk with people at the gym or a park

So instead of replying, "I'm a dentist," what should you say? It depends on what you have to offer that's interesting… and different. It could be:

- "I'm a dentist on the west side of town. We do veneers, whitening and keep up to date on all types of cosmetic treatment. And we see families as well."
- "I help people replace missing teeth without full dentures or partial dentures so they can confidently eat the foods they enjoy and improve their appearance."
- "I see adults who want the very finest dentistry delivered in a relaxed and comfortable environment."

Your elevator speech is similar to branding which is why it's essential to say what is unique and exciting about your practice… what makes you better than the competition. Even though the Elevator Speech is memorized, it should sound off the cuff.

Take a few minutes and create your elevator speech. Be sure to include information that differentiates your practice and will pique the person's interest. Then repeat it until it sounds natural.

Remember, case acceptance is a series of conversations you have with people… even conversations in elevators. So always be thinking, "What's the next step in the series, and how can I influence that step to occur right now?" As an example, before the elevator door opens, hand the person your business card and invite them to visit your website; or come to the office for a complimentary, preliminary exam.

When it comes right down to it, every public action you take is marketing. Even riding in elevators.

123 Average Lifetime Value

There are some practice management dollar figures that are deceptively important for you to know. One of those is the Average Lifetime Value (ALV) of an implant patient. First, I'll explain how to calculate an ALV. Then, I'll explain how to use this information.

Calculating Your ALV

Let's say implant patients invest an average of $12,000 the first year they're in your practice. Then they are with you for an average of 10 years spending an average of $600 a year. The ALV for this patient is $12,000 + $,6000 = $18,000. It's reasonable to assume that this patient would refer at least one other implant patient over those 10 years. So $18,000 plus a second $18,000 equals $36,000. Some practices will have a lower implant ALV. Some will be higher. Calculate your ALV now.

Using Your ALV

Now that you know your ALV, you can use it as a yardstick to help you answer two very important practice management questions:

1. How much time and money should I invest to attract implant patients?
2. How much time and money should I invest to keep them?

ATTRACT THEM – Let's say you build a marketing program that attracts 12 implant patients a year. Twelve implant patients times a $36,000 ALV equals $540,000 revenue into your practice over 11 years. How much would you invest in marketing to bring in $540K? I know an individual dentist who spends over $40K a year on implant marketing. I don't know your practice's financial figures or your position on the path to implant excellence. So I can't tell you what your figure should be. Only your financial advisor and you can do that.

KEEP THEM – When treated fantastically and communicated with well, these $540K ALV patients will become loyal patients. They will accept your treatment recommendations without question. They may move away, but fly back twice a year for their recare visits. They will refer not just one patient over 10 years, but one or two patients a year. In my book, *Implant Excellence,* I give you dozens of unique ways to connect and communicate with these patients so they are with you for a lifetime.

Pull the *Implant Excellence* book off your shelf now. Reread the marketing information now because… repetition is the mother of all skills.

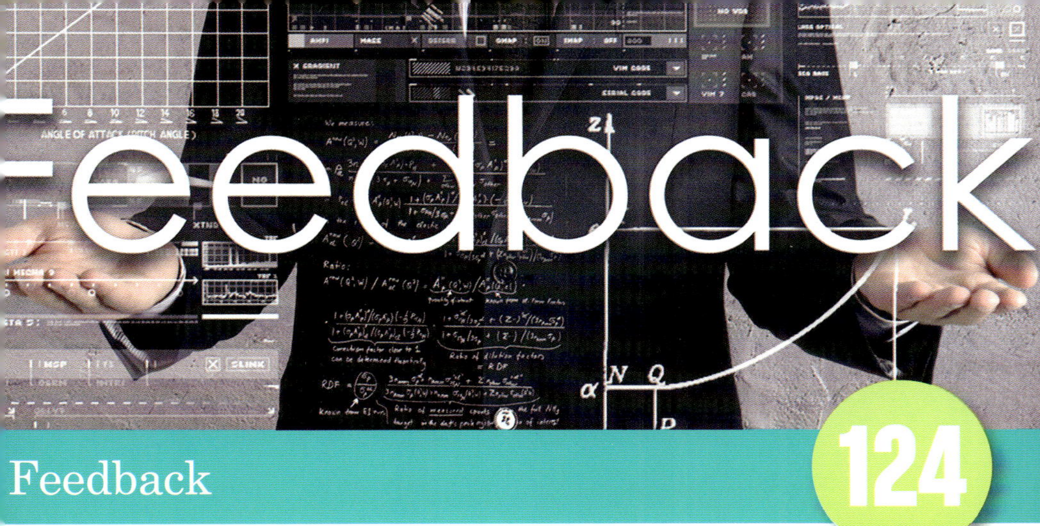

Feedback

124

The worst feedback is no feedback. And that is what most dentists receive. In their efforts to avoid negative remarks and unfulfilled expectations, these dentists hide from feedback by not soliciting it or act in ways that minimize its impact.

I know there are automated ways to receive this information, but it's not nearly as effective as face-to-face feedback. Here are two times you can do this:

1. When patients express dissatisfaction – Ask them what happened to create the dissatisfaction. Get specific answers so you can implement specific remedies.
2. On a routine basis – Have your treatment care coordinator (See my Implant Excellence book) or office manager sit down with patients at their final restorative appointments and have the following conversation:

   You: "Maria, we value you as a patient and a person and respect your ideas. Would you mind if I ask you a couple of questions concerning your experience with us?"

   Maria: "Not at all."

   You: "Great. What are one or two things we do extremely well?"

   Maria: "You do A, B and C well."

   You: "Thanks. I'll make sure I mention that to Donna. Anything else?"

   Maria: "Can't think of anything."

   You: "What is one thing we could do better?"

   Maria: "Well, you could…"

   You: "Excellent feedback. What else could we improve?"

   Maria: "That's all I can think of."

   You: "Thanks for your feedback. I'll make sure we address your one concern."

After you receive feedback, make sure it's put to good use. Discuss feedback at a team meeting, or have a personal conversation with a team member who's struggling. Feedback + Action = Practice Improvement. I know it's easier not to put this formula into play. But trust me, it'll be worth it.

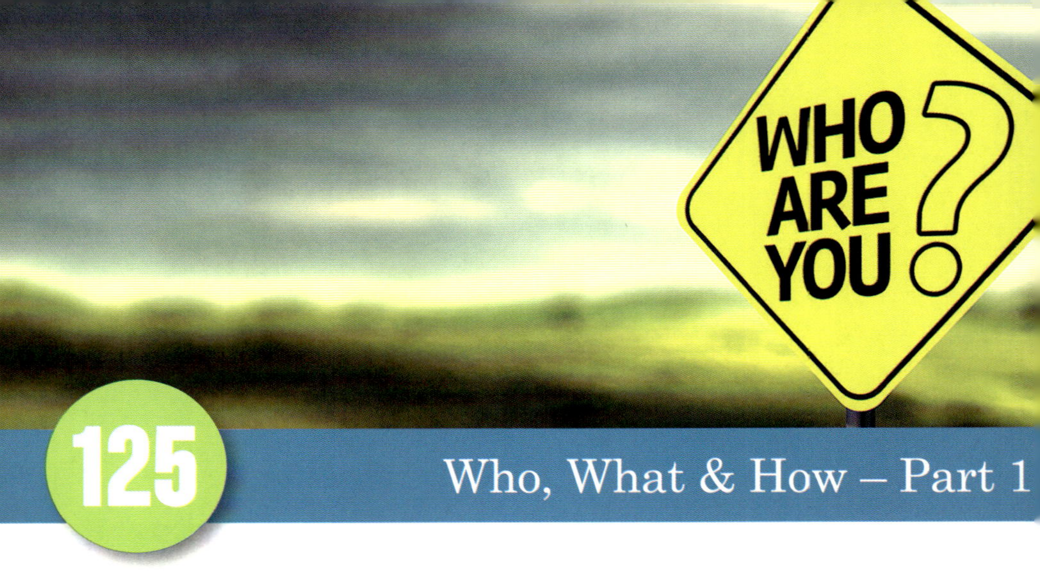

125 Who, What & How – Part 1

The best marketing campaigns dramatically deliver one or more of the following three messages:

- **Who You Are**
- **What You Do**
- **How You Do It**

The first message, "Who You Are," conveys nothing about your training, the quality of your dentistry or your service. It tells the more powerful story of the person you truly are. The time-honored saying, "People don't care how much you know until they know how much you care," applies here.

Here's an example of message #1 in action. I have a friend who wanted facial cosmetic surgery. She interviewed three surgeons. The first one had the best reputation in the area with fees to match. The person had a lavish office with a gorgeous and stylishly dressed team and was very friendly and knowledgeable in the interview.

The second surgeon had an excellent reputation with above average fees. His office was beautifully decorated and his team was well dressed and courteous. Like the first surgeon, he was friendly and knowledgeable.

The third surgeon had an excellent reputation with average fees. His office was nice, but not ritzy. His team was casually dressed and friendly. In the interview, the third surgeon was cordial, relaxed and spent a little more time with my friend talking about non-surgical topics including his philanthropic interests and places he'd visited.

My friend chose the third surgeon. Why? Because of who he was. Not because of his experience, surgical reputation or fancy office.

Here are some questions for you:

1. Do you have an emotional "Who I am" message to convey? If not, how will you create one? You can't fake it here. People can spot a phony a mile away. Almost all "Who I am" professional messages involve you giving to others.
2. How will you convey your message with internal marketing, external marketing and public relations? Internal marketing (the surgeon's calendar) and public relations (free PR in your community) are naturals for telling "Who I am" stories.

In the next tips, I'll discuss the "What You Do" message. Until then, be a person who cares about others outside the office. Everyone will benefit.

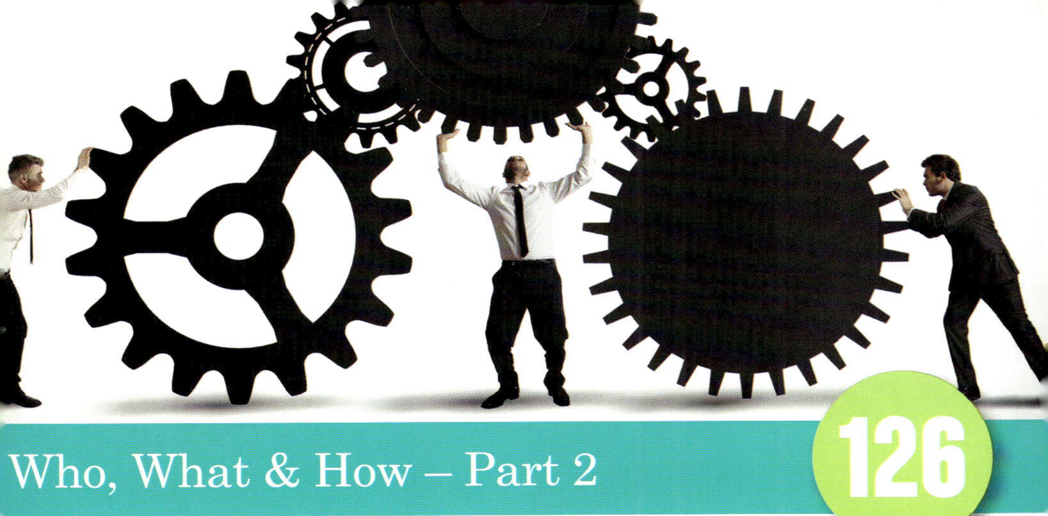

Who, What & How – Part 2

"What You Do" isn't what it seems. "What You Do" is not the actions you take (placing restorations or restoring implants). It is the value you provide your patients from their perspective. The value comes in two forms:

1. The pain alleviated
2. The pleasure provided

Here's an example of what I mean. I know a dentist who knows exactly what he does. He positively changes people's lives. His entire marketing campaign centers around the theme: **Change Your Smile. Change Your Life**. His radio commercials are his patients telling listeners how cosmetic dentistry changed their smiles and...changed their lives. His magazine and newspaper ads do the same.

Many of my students place and restore implants that help people throw away their floating lower dentures (relieve pain) and receive ones that snap into place. Now they can talk with confidence and eat the food they love (provide pleasure). I have another colleague who built a state-of-the-art practice in rural Wisconsin where people could obtain the pleasure of "high quality dentistry right here in southwest Wisconsin" so they don't have to travel to the big cities to receive the best that dentistry has to offer.

Some dentists diagnose and treat sleep apnea so their patients drastically reduce a major health risk, sleep better and don't disturb their bed partners. Talk about reducing pain and providing pleasure.

I have two questions for you: What do you do? And is your message describing it in an impactful way? Your answers will go a long way to predicting your practice's success and your patients' levels of pleasure.

In my next Tips, I'll discuss the "How You Do It" message. Until then, don't just do dentistry. Change people's lives.

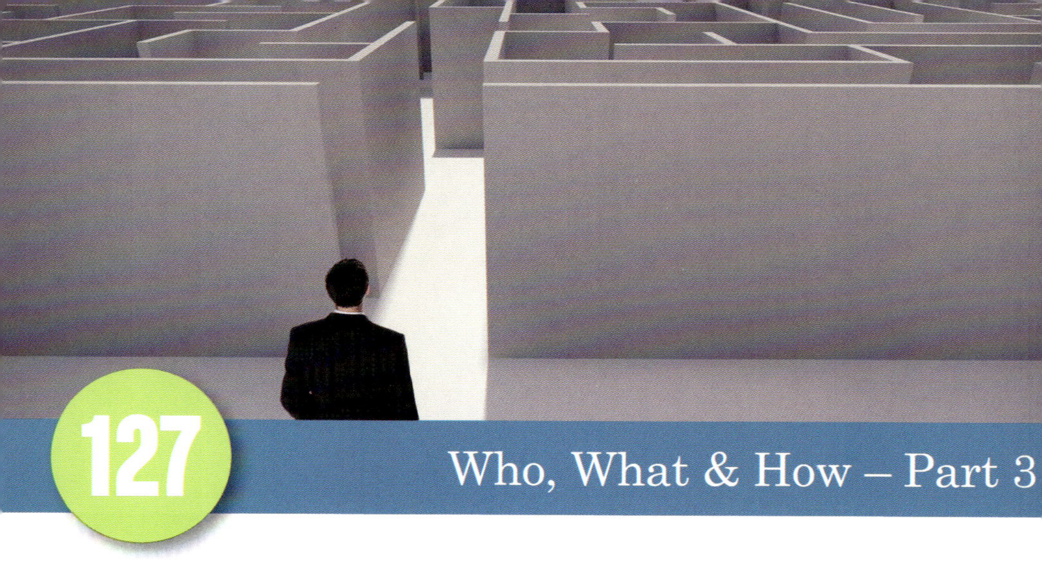

127 Who, What & How – Part 3

In a nutshell, "How You Do It" is the experience you wrap around your dental care. Here's an example of what I'm talking about. With almost zero advertising, Hershey sells three million chocolate Kisses a day! How do they pull that off? Is it the quality of the chocolate? No way. Hershey has discovered something all dentists need to know. People want experiences.

I believe that all business (including dentistry) is show business. Why does Johnnie Depp make around $30 million per movie while PhD college professors earn $110,000 per year? He's in show business and makes people feel fantastic as they watch his movies. The professor educates. Why are 20 of the world's 27 largest hotels in Las Vegas? Because Las Vegas is entertaining to millions; and each hotel is a different experience.

In addition to providing high-quality care, I believe your dental office needs to be in the experience business too by focusing on all five senses: sight, sound, touch, smell and taste. Now can you see why Hershey sells three million Kisses a day? They create a memorable experience with every Kiss.

- Sight - Every uniquely shaped Kiss is wrapped in silver foil with a pull-string on top.
- Sound – A special sound is made as you pull the string and pop open the Kiss.
- Touch – The silver wrapping has a unique feel. The Kiss has a yummy feel in your mouth.
- Smell – The chocolate smells good.
- Taste – The chocolate tastes even better than it should because all five of your senses have been positively activated.

Once a year, your entire team needs to walk in your patients' shoes. Start in the parking lot. Pay attention to all five senses. Which positive ones can you enhance? Which negative ones can you eliminate or reduce? Now walk through the door and sit in the reception area. Does any of the sensory input need a tune-up? Now lie in a hygiene and clinical chair. Do this while real patients are in the office to get a realistic experience. How do those ceiling tiles look? Look at, touch, taste and smell all the gadgets and gizmos you typically put in patients' mouths. Can you find products that create a better experience?

Be like a Hershey's Kiss, Johnnie Depp and Las Vegas. Focus on How You Do It. Create memorable experiences for your patients using all five senses. Your patients will appreciate it and your entire team will have the thrill of being in show business.

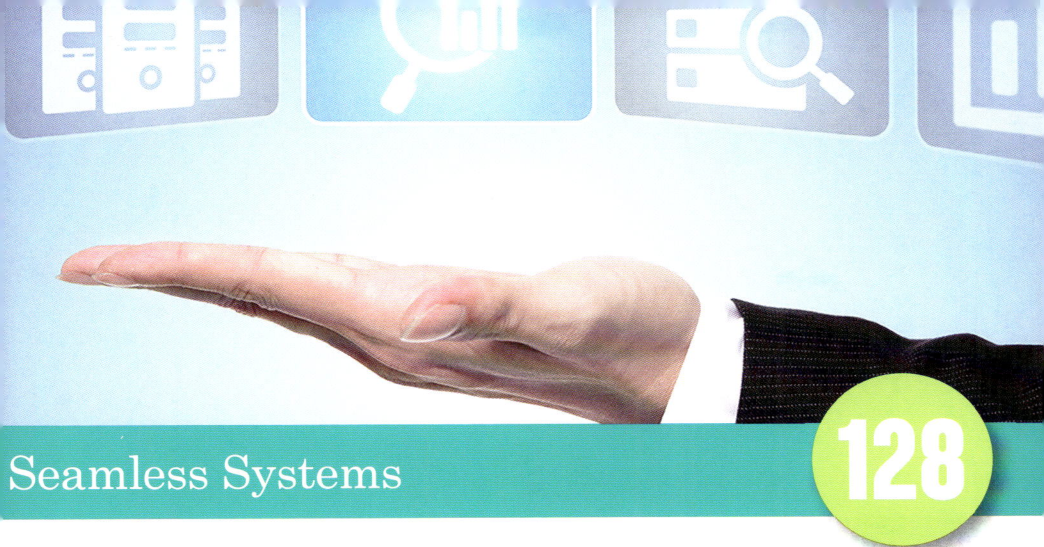

Seamless Systems

128

In the 1990 television commercial for the LifeCall medical alert pendent, the elderly Mrs. Fletcher fell in her bathroom. She proceeded to activate her alarm and tell the dispatcher, "I've fallen, and I can't get up."

A similar situation occurs with many dentists' marketing efforts. They have a system in play, but the system has one or more seams in it. When prospective patients come to the seam, they trip over it, fall down and can't get up.

Here are five places these seams could appear in marketing:

1. A dentist does a terrific job with search engine optimization (SEO), search engine marketing (SEM) and/or pay per click marketing, but when patients go to their website, the site doesn't influence them to take the next step. And the next step isn't always Call for an Appointment.
2. Patients call the office, but the person answering the phone doesn't have the skills to effectively influence callers to take the next step. Or you have an office policy in place that discourages complimentary Meet & Greet visits where your Patient Care Coordinator or you assess their situations and have a brief consultation with them.
3. The dentist doesn't have the skills needed to accurately diagnose comprehensive dentistry.
4. The dentist's team doesn't have the skills or the time to conduct a series of conversations with patients to elegantly influence them to take action on treatment recommendations.
5. The dentist doesn't have the skills needed to complete comprehensive dentistry.

Seams can pop up in any sequence of events in your office. Common problem sequences include:

- Scheduling
- Records and bookkeeping
- Leadership and management
- Supplies
- Laboratory coordination

Sometimes dentists are so close to their situations that they don't even see the seams right in front of their eyes. That why it's important to periodically have an outsider do seam checks on your practice's systems.

Don't let gaps in your systems prevent patients from receiving the care they desire and deserve. Mrs. Fletcher may have fallen, but your patients and your practice deserve to stand tall.

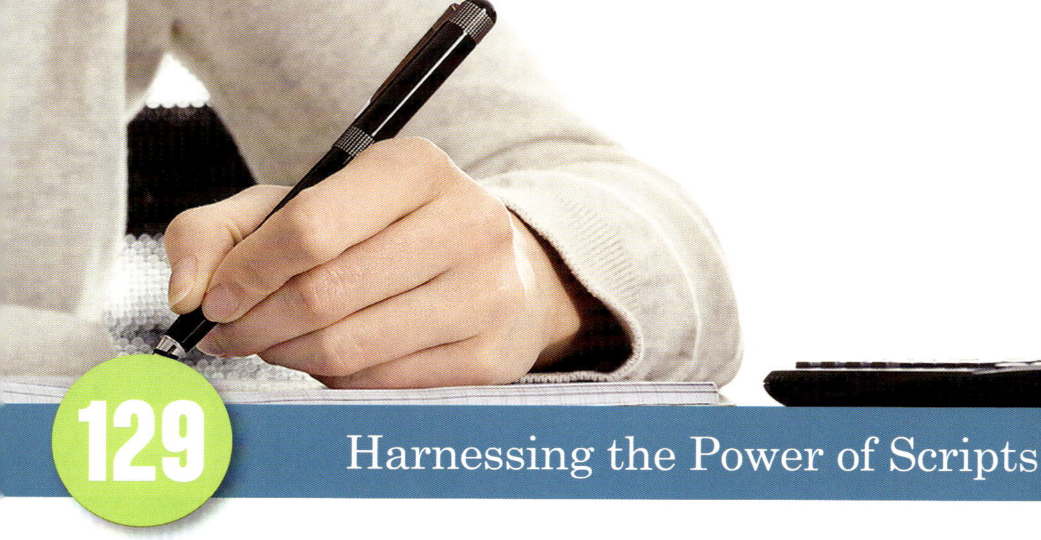

129 Harnessing the Power of Scripts

I think scripts are great. But for the scripts to have real power, the user must own the words. If you ask someone to say a script they don't believe in or that doesn't feel comfortable, you're shooting them (and yourself) in the foot. They won't use the script because it's too painful to do so. Or they will use the script (say the right words), but betray the message by being incongruent. People are incongruent when their words deliver one message and their voice qualities and body language deliver a different message.

Here is the 10-step process I'd recommend for harnessing the power of scripts:

- Precisely determine the outcome you want to create from the script. If you don't know where you're going, any road will get you there.
- Review two or three sample scripts for ideas.
- Write the script in conversational language.
- Read the script out loud. Based on what you hear, revise the script.
- Make sure the people using the script agree and feel comfortable with it.
- If not, have them rewrite the script in their own words while retaining the full meaning of the original.
- Check the new script and agree with the content.
- Have the people practice the script in private.
- Have them role-play with another team member until the words naturally roll out of their mouths.
- Have them use it in the real world.

One of the first rules of leadership is "Decide what's important and talk about it over and over." Effective communication with your patients is definitely important. That's why your scripts should be an important part of your policies and procedures manual.

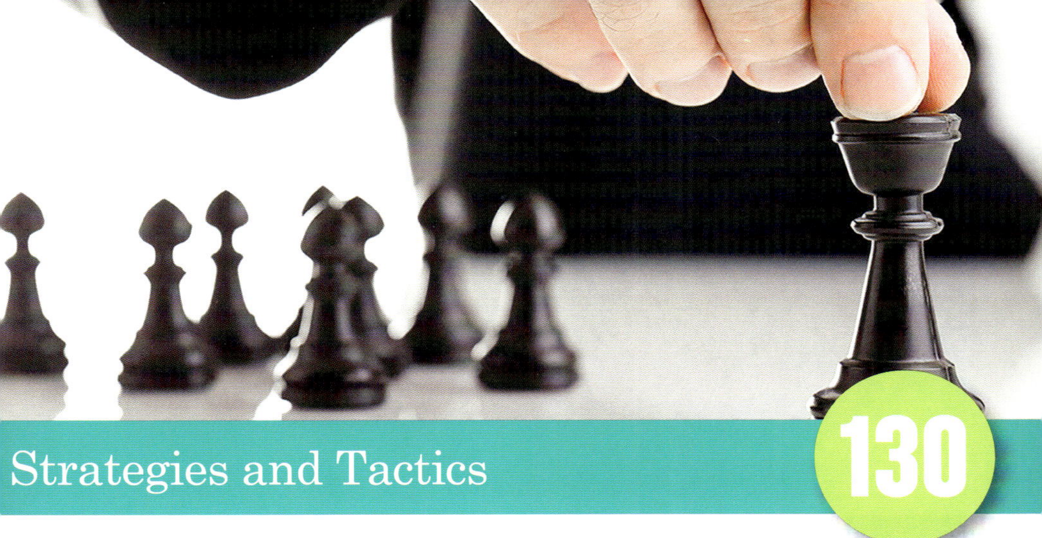

Strategies and Tactics

130

Strategies are big and invisible to all but the strategy creator. They are the all-encompassing plans you have to achieve important goals. Tactics are small and easily seen. They are the individual actions that make the strategies work.

Most dentists are tactical. This means they do more of the same activities and work harder. Successful dentists create effective strategies first. Then they focus on tactics. The result? They work smarter.

Here's an example of strategic thinking. What do you want to have happen on a call from someone interested in your practice? This is another way of saying, "What are your strategic objectives for taking an inbound call from a prospect?" Think of two or three strategic objectives right now.

If you're having challenges coming up with answers, it may be a sign you need to think more strategically. There are no universally right or wrong answers. It depends on your type of practice and your goals. Here is a list of possible strategic objectives:

- Connect with the caller. Strengthen rapport and trust.
- Gather basic information.
- Qualify the caller. What are their problems and desires? Maybe they would be better served in another practice. If so, you want to discover this ASAP.
- Motivate the person to take action quicker.
- Intrigue the caller by making a connection between what she wants and what you can deliver. As an example, if she mentions interest in implants, say, "Elle, you've called the right practice. The doctor is an implant expert and has extensive implant training."
- Determine the best next step and influence her to take it.

Now that I've given you some examples, write your top 2–4 strategic objectives for taking an inbound call from a prospective patient.

To achieve those objectives, will that change the set of tactics you use? Will it change:

- Who is answering the phone?
- What they say?
- How they say what they say?
- The questions they ask?
- The direction they steer the conversation?
- What is agreed to at the end of the call?

There are many factors that lead to the practice of your dreams. Strategies first and tactics second is one of the most important.

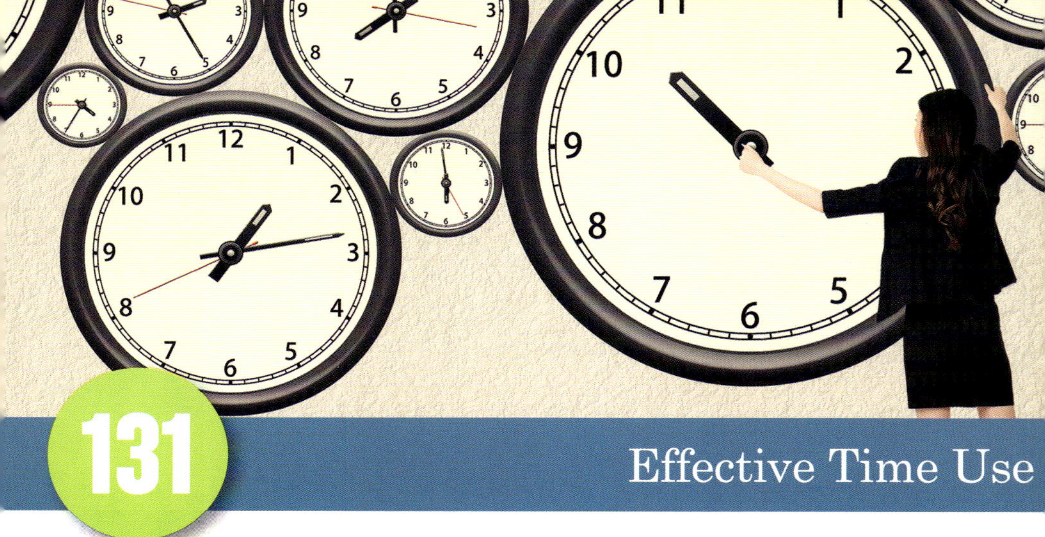

131 Effective Time Use

You're feeling overwhelmed. You have clinical dentistry to complete, a practice to run, a family to support and a life to live. You say to yourself, "If only I had more time!" Well, you've got all the time there is. So that can't be the problem. The challenge is to use your time effectively.

Understanding the difference between important activities and urgent activities is an essential time management skill. Important activities have outcomes that lead to personal or professional achievement. Urgent activities demand your immediate attention. Important activities may or may not be urgent.

An example of an important activity that is urgent is seeing the patients on your schedule. Examples of important activities that are not urgent are training, planning and relationship building. Because these three are important, but not urgent, you must put them into your schedule first. Then hold yourself accountable for doing them. If not, the urgencies in your day will always crowd them out.

Below are three scheduling steps that will help you maximize your time:

- Keeping in mind your important and urgent activities, put the important but not urgent activities into your schedule first. In addition to training, planning and relationship building activities. This category includes spending time with your spouse and/or kids, exercising and doing hobbies.
- Now schedule your important and urgent activities. In addition to seeing patients, this category includes attending important business, family and personal obligations.
- Spend the time you have left doing activities that are not important. These include most phone calls, needless meetings, useless Internet surfing, TV watching and other time wasters. Be careful of filling your day with activities that are important to others, but not you. Politely saying, "No," is the best way to handle these requests.

Fill your daily time bucket with the activities that are important to you. If you don't take control over this vital activity, your schedule will fill up with nonessentials and will lead to a life that is unfulfilled.

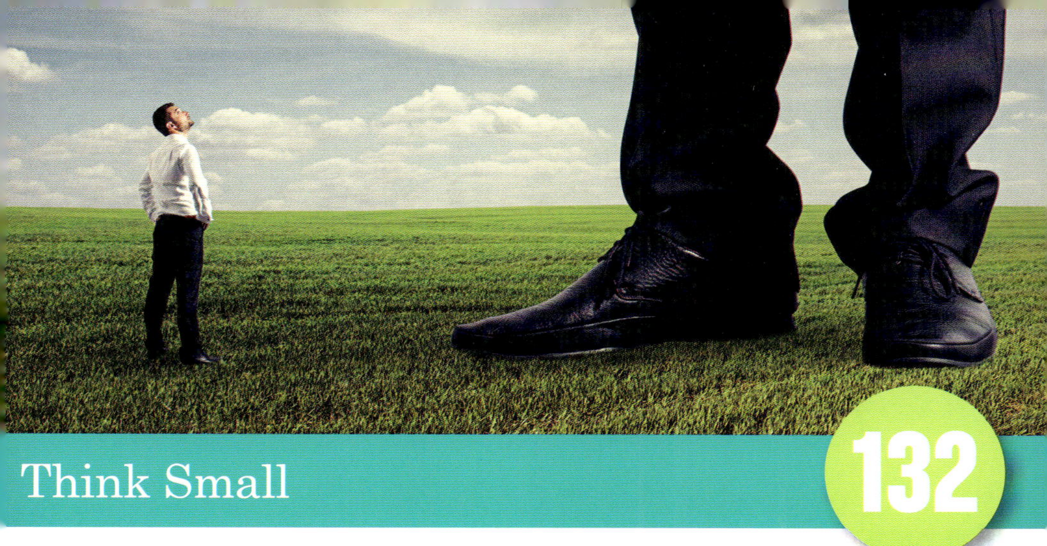

Think Small

132

The big picture also shows that only 66% of the U.S. population visits a dental office annually. The big picture also shows that most people only want to do what their dental insurance covers or only restore a tooth when it needs to be fixed.

If you're the ADA, General Motors or a presidential candidate, "big" matters. If you need over 50% of the population to make your numbers, you have to pay attention to the big picture. But most dentists only want 100 to 200 new patients a year, not 100,000.

When you pay exclusive attention to the "big," you're playing a numbers game and treating the market as if it's a gigantic ball of sameness. But the entire market is not what your market is. Your market is the smaller group of people who want the types and quality of dentistry you deliver.

Here's an example of what I mean. Let's assume you want to increase the number of implants you place and restore. Let's also assume there are 100,000 adults in your area; and that 60,000 of them have missing teeth. Finally, let's assume that only 6,000 have the financial resources and interest to replace these missing teeth with implants. One hundred thousand and 60,000 are really big numbers. If you focus on attracting the whole group of 100,000 or even the 60,000 then:

- It won't work out because what you deliver is not what the masses desire.
- You will lose effectiveness with the 6,000 you want as patients because you're trying to be all things to all people. And sameness is not what the 6,000 desire. They want implant expertise.

The great thing is that these 6,000 people tend to use the internet to research topics important to them. They tend to read certain local magazines. This means they can be relatively easy to communicate with.

Consider these questions:

- Do you use pay per click, search engine optimization and search engine marketing to attract these folks?
- Do you advertise in or write educational articles for the periodicals they read?
- Is your community reputation one that appeals to this small group?
- Are you thinking big and losing impact with the groups you want to attract?

To most dentists, micro groups matter more than macro ones. But most of all, people matter. Individual human beings with unique names, wants and interests. When you serve them well, you will be served in return.

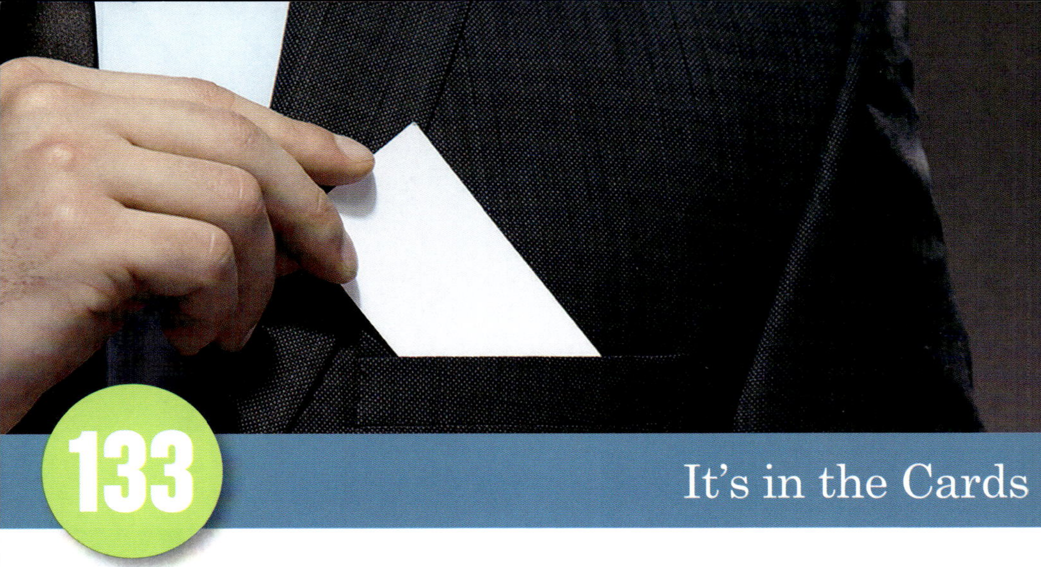

133 It's in the Cards

One effective marketing action you can take right now is to make sure every team member and you carry a few business cards. When you're at a grocery store, bank, gym, hair salon, dry cleaner, gas station, restaurant or office supply store, you can hand them out to people you meet.

Your business cards should be much more than your name, address and telephone number. In addition, put your web address, facebook info and other social media information on the card. Use both sides of the card. A personal note written on the back greatly increases the odds the person will keep the card and record its information.

If you really want to make a positive impression with tech savvy people, have a Quick Response Code (QR Code) on the back of your cards. People who have a QR Code app installed on their smartphones can take a photo of your code. The phone will automatically convert the image into a URL directing the phone's browser to your practice's website.

At select times, you can also wear your business card. When your team and you are out in the community, wear your office scrubs. It's a bonus when your office logo and name tag is also visible. This means having clean, spare clinical attire used for outside the office only. You would be amazed how many people will come up to you and ask dental-related questions or where your office is located. When they do, give them a big smile and your card.

Many offices provide financial rewards when new patients mention they received a business card from team members. I know one woman who made an extra $700 last year by influencing 35 people to schedule visits to her office. The best part of that story is that everyone benefits – the patient, the team member and your bottom line.

I totally agree with the premise of Fred Joyal's fantastic book, Everything Is Marketing. The correct use of your paper and clothing business cards is an important part of your marketing campaign… and inexpensive. Use them often and well.

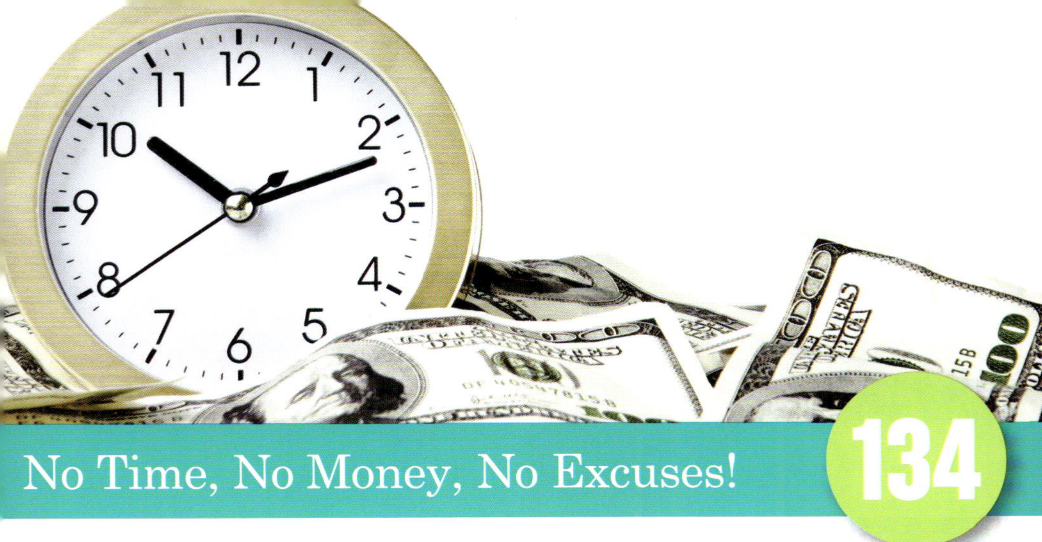

No Time, No Money, No Excuses!

134

Be honest, what are your top excuses for not getting something done or not tending to task? I'll give you 30 seconds. Ready. Go!

Chances are "there's not enough time" and "there's not enough money" ranked high on your list.

In business these are two of the most common.

Consider how often in your dental practice you've delayed an important conversation, ignored a pressing problem, or deferred a big decision like purchasing a new CBCT scanner or enrolling in a continuing education course "for another day." This is an instinctual response – rooted in our early Hominid fight for survival. Who cared about long-term planning when animals needed to be hunted for food and the fire needed to be lit? In that do-or-die era, tomorrow could wait.

Except that it couldn't. At least not really.

If our ancestors were only focused on the here and now, the long-term planning skills needed to develop language, civilization, currency, culture and art, wouldn't have been realized.

The fact is, there is enough time. We all have the same 24 hours in a day. (And at Earth's current rate of decreasing rotation we'll have a 25-hour day in 140 million years.) It's just how we use it that matters most. The same holds true for money. As money is the medium through which the value of goods and services is expressed, money is shorthand for those same hunter-gatherer necessities.

There always seems to be enough money to survive when times are tough. The trick is to plan for tomorrow – to allocate resources after immediate needs have been met.

Dental practice ownership, like life, can be difficult. But the more "bread" (money) you got, the more those difficulties can be blunted.

Review your list of top excuses. And if you do nothing else after reading this book, delete "there's no time," and "there's no money."

There is time. And there is money. Use them correctly and your dental practice will prosper!

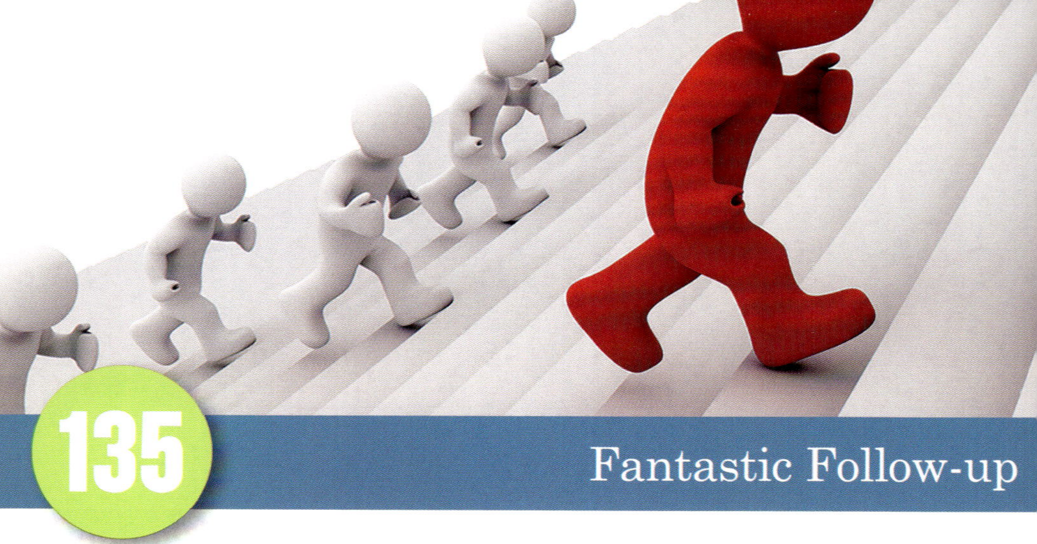

135 Fantastic Follow-up

When it comes to practice success, many dentists are their own worst enemies. They want to grow, but they never take the time or make the effort. And they miss simple marketing opportunities staring them right in the face.

Here's an example of what I mean. A few months ago a friend of mine upgraded his home stereo system. When installed, the system and the service were excellent. So what's the problem? He was never contacted by the shop after the sale to see if there was another location (like his office) that could use a similar enhancement. I'm sure if this shop worked to get another sale from a satisfied customer, without doing anything else, their business would increase by at least 20%.

When was the last time the people who fitted you with glasses followed up to see if you wanted a spare pair of sunglasses with the new prescription? Probably never. If they made that a regular practice, their business would also increase significantly.

How about the restaurants, dry cleaners or hair salons you frequent? Do they stay in touch and attempt to get additional sales from you? I doubt it. Instead, they spend their time and money chasing after new customers.

Does your dental practice fall into the same category? If so, begin regularly communicating with your patients and influencing them to accept needed and wanted dental care. It's vitally important to your practice's success. Keep your existing patients happy, interested, and asking for more.

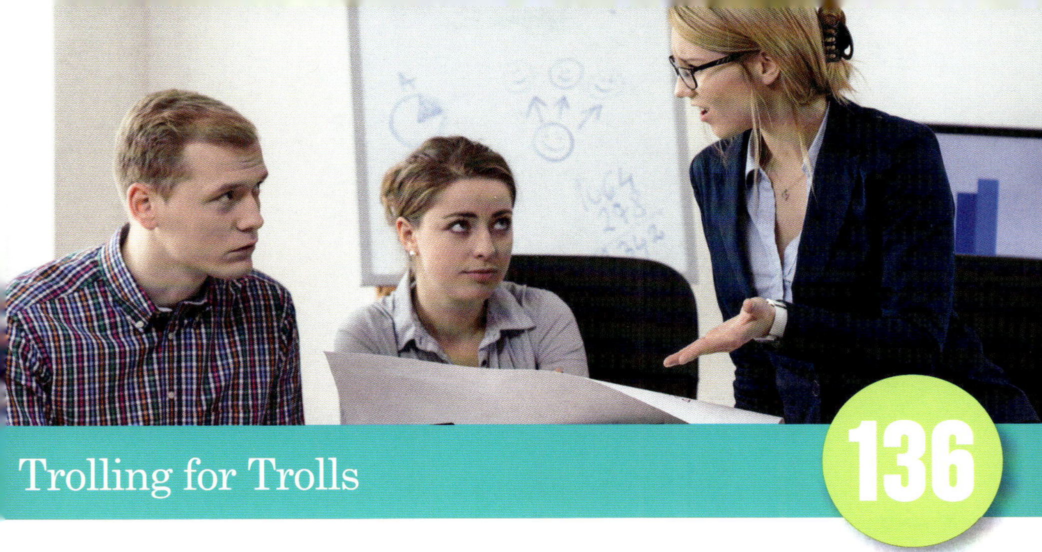

Trolling for Trolls

136

Despite the most rigorous hiring standards, despite the personal oversight of each member brought on board, despite impeccable resumes and job histories, despite all of this, organizations will invariably hire a meeting troll.

Meeting trolls thrive on cultivating negativity. While the unskilled troll might resort to blatant undermining, more typical is the subtle approach. At face value many of their concerns are justified.

But the tone is what sets these people apart.

A critique of a new policy or program is more than justified. A laundry list of constant complaints complete with negative body language and no suggested solutions or modifications to these plans is not.

When the meeting is over, you can be sure the proverbial water cooler talk has already begun. Office chitchat, via text, email and private messaging apps has already begun. Over time, such dissention in the ranks can undermine your leadership.

Fortunately dental offices are businesses not prone to having lengthy – or frequent – meetings. But as other tips have noted, having more of them, especially if they iron out concrete goals, isn't a bad thing.

So the meeting troll might have gone undetected in your organization for years.

Once a meeting troll has been identified, the next step is resolving the issue.

I suggest a multistep approach. Begin gently. Speak to the offending individual outside office hours or during lunch and express your concerns about their meeting behavior. Here, the "sandwich method" is particularly popular. Start with a compliment, then offer your criticism, and close the discussion with another compliment, or at least a lighter tone.

For example:

"Mark, I really appreciate the time and effort you put in to offering your points of view in our monthly meetings. However, I would appreciate suggested solutions to the criticisms you raise. Doing so will inspire the whole team, and it will inspire me!"

Depending on how Mark responds to this opening salvo will dictate your next response.

It's never easy confronting meeting trolls. But the sooner you do, the healthier your dental practice will be.

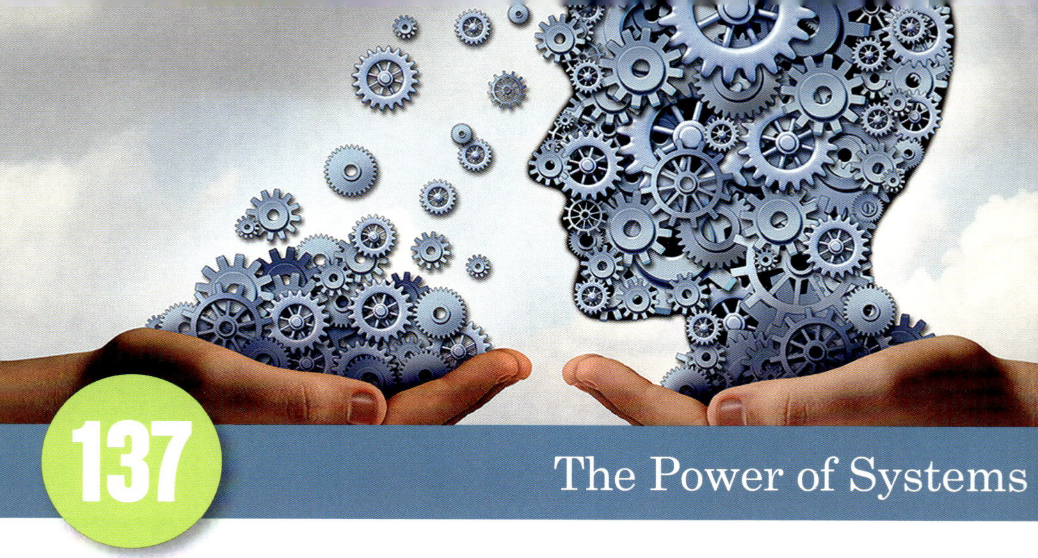

137 The Power of Systems

There are three factors leading to successful dental practice implementation that I see in the hundreds of dentists I work with each year:

1. Motivation
2. Skills
3. Systems

Implementing any change in your office may be simple, but it's probably not going to be easy. This is why your team and you must be motivated to consistently take action through time… even when the going gets tough.

By itself, motivation is not enough because people who are just motivated, but don't know what they're doing, are dangerous. You must have the clinical, practice management, communication and relationship skills needed to succeed.

You can be the most motivated group in the world… with fantastic levels of skill in every important area, but you won't implement successfully unless you have a system that puts your skills into play in the right order, at the right time, in the right way.

If you watched Super Bowl XLVII, you saw two extremely motivated teams composed of players with top-notch skills. Did you notice that both teams had different, but very effective, offensive, defensive and special systems they used to harness the power of their players' skills? And that the systems they used fit the unique skills of the players on their rosters? The Baltimore Ravens' quarterback would have been a failure in San Francisco's offensive system… and vice versa.

So what are your skills as a dentist and a person? What are the skills of your current team members? And have you created the systems needed to harness the power of everyone's skills? If not, you may experience considerable frustration. You're motivated. You're skillful. But your systems aren't the right ones for you.

So how do you locate and implement the best systems? Just like NFL football teams do… by seeing what is working with other teams and then adapting those systems to their personnel. And by innovating every once in a while with something that has never been done. Doing this isn't simple… or easy. But the challenge is worth it! Just ask the Ravens.

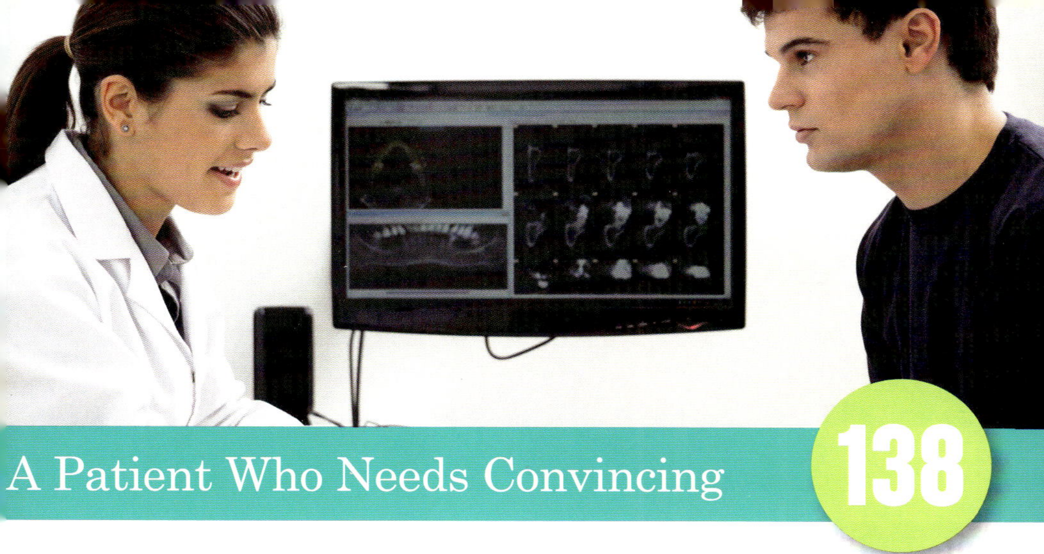

A Patient Who Needs Convincing

Here's a basic marketing fact every dental practice owner should know: the more real you make your product to the patient, the more convincing its purchase or use becomes.

It's a bit disheartening when you think about it. So many of your patients dread coming to the dentist – even for procedures designed to transform their lives like teeth whitening, cosmetic smile makeovers, and orthodontics.

You have to walk in their shoes. From their perspective, any dental visit is a type of medical checkup. Dental visits are expensive, sometimes painful or mildly unpleasant, and for many, anxiety inducing.

This is where your salesmanship capabilities can really shine. How well are you selling the *image* of what you're promoting?

Marketing gurus suggest two approaches. Engage the five senses (or at least evoke later use of the five senses) and use emotions to connect with your patients.

Here's an example:

Decades of research confirm the obvious: the perfect smile is a pathway to success.

- Imagine that third round job interview that concludes with a strong handshake and a healthy, natural, confident smile.
- See yourself at the party becoming the social butterfly you always knew was trapped inside.
- Make a lasting impression on a first date.

Warm, genuine smiles are an essential ingredient to our effect on others. Don't delay in giving your confidence the smile it deserves!

If financing is a concern, offer your own anecdotes about how either you or another patient faced similar concerns. And that together you worked out a payment solution that was agreeable to all parties.

Will all patients that need convincing ultimately go for it?

No.

But being passionate about what you're offering, and genuine in your desire to help transform their lives will turn Nays into Yays.

Convinced yet?!?

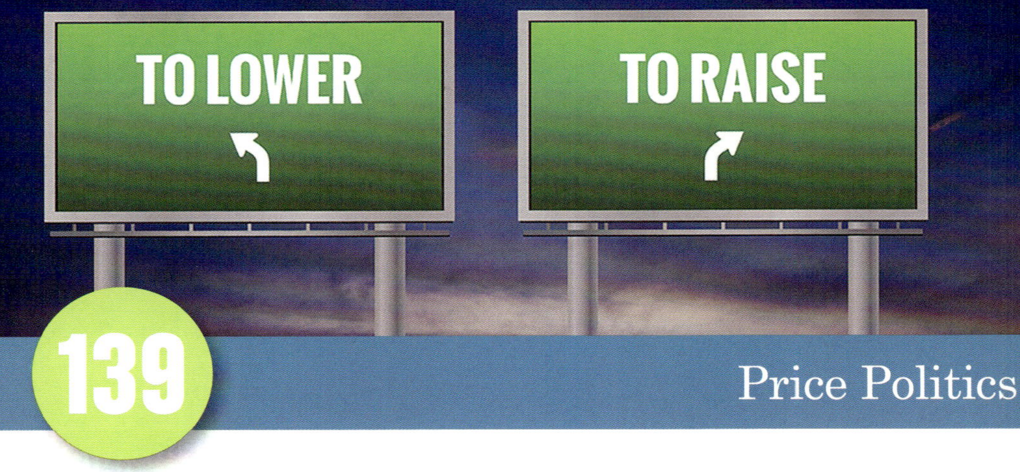

139 Price Politics

Question – What's the total worth of the services you offer your patients?

Answer – Whatever a patient is willing to pay for it.

While the above might seem a little off-putting, the answer speaks to the basic economic principle of Value.

And it's true. At a fundamental level, the value of something is always relative to the buyer. Everyone's needs are unique; therefore the specific utility they receive from a purchase differs.

Of course following this logic to its ultimate conclusion is unwise. Essentially it means the return to bartering. Every price is haggled. Every item's value is unique and constantly in flux depending on the needs of the merchant and customer.

But in a complex society, price standardization and thereby value standardization is equally important. Imagine how difficult it would be if the price you paid at the pump varied by how urgently you needed gas, or your car's fuel efficiency? Chaos – or at least absurdly long lines and a lot of wasted fuel spent idling – would be the result.

Your dental practice needs to balance these extremes as well. While price standardization is a boon to your accounting department, hyper rigidity and an inflexibility to work with patients who value your services, but struggle affording the care, could backfire. It's important to work with all patients and find ways to accommodate their financial needs.

Of course, you have to have limits. But don't play price politics with your patients either.

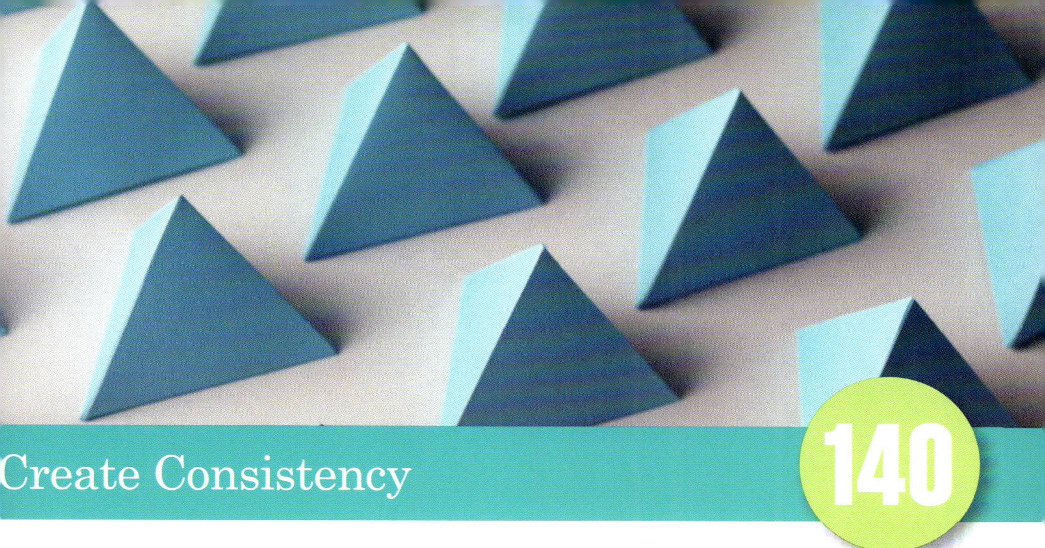

Create Consistency

140

Zagat, the company that evaluates restaurants across the country, released its latest ratings of fast-food chains. McDonald's was the winner in many categories? Surprised? Ever go to an airport or mall food court and notice the longest line is at McDonald's? It happens all the time even though some of the other choices are more unique like local restaurants.

Most people would agree that Mickey D's doesn't serve fantastic food. But one thing they do offer is consistency. Consistency is a vital factor missing in many dental practices. And this inconsistency is costing them big time.

Here are some areas where I see inconsistency in dental practices:

1. Telephone conversations – especially those conversations with people calling for the first time
2. Responses to patient questions – team members don't have the information they need, so they wing it or say, "I don't know"
3. First visit examination – it's done differently based on how much time the dentist and/or hygienist have that day
4. Case presentation – it's squeezed between clinical procedures and frequently gets short-changed
5. Clinical philosophies – especially when dentists and hygienists have varying philosophies of periodontal care

To improve the consistency in your practice, remember these three words: standards, inspection and training.

1. **Standards** - You must set your standards high in every area of your practice.
2. **Inspection** - Inspect your team's behavior to make sure the standards are upheld. People will respect what you inspect.
3. **Training** - Train your team so they know exactly what to do and how to do it. Now everyone will do it the same way.

Being inconsistent in your practice creates confusion among your patients and team. And it wastes time and money. Every team member (including you) has to be on the same page when it comes to all procedures in your practice. It's the "secret sauce" that makes McDonald's number one. It will do the same for your practice.

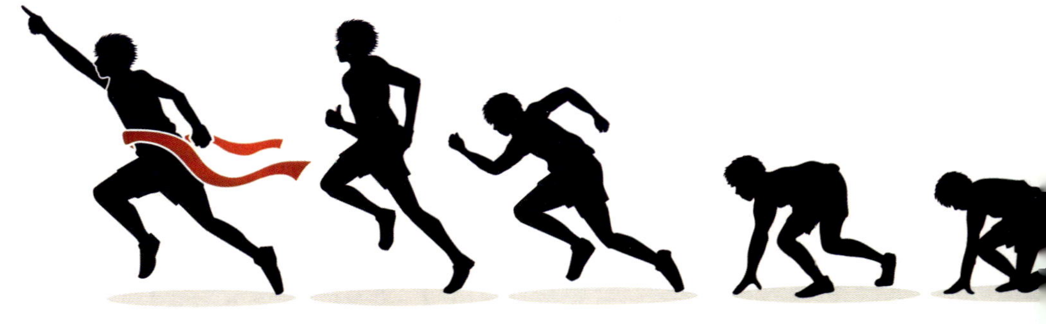

141 Sprint vs. Endurance

Most people, even non-athletes, know that there are two types of basic runs: the sprint and the endurance run.

A sprint is when a runner runs at their top speed for a short burst. In case you're wondering, Mike Boit, of Kenya, who ran a mile in 3 minutes 28 seconds in 1983, holds the world record (for the downhill mile)! An endurance run is a lower, slower, test of stamina.

These are your marathon runners – the pavement pounders who carefully conserve energy for the many miles ahead. Some miles are run faster than others. It's all about strategy.

Businesses must think like this too.

While it might be tempting to launch your dental practice at full tilt in the beginning, it helps to think like a marathon runner. A marathon runner has 26.2 miles in front of them at the starting line. A dental practice owner just starting out may have 26 years in front of them – maybe more.

When building your practice from the ground up, it helps to keep the long game in mind. Save your strength. Conserve your mental fortitude. It's easy to be over zealous.

Think endurance, *not sprint!*

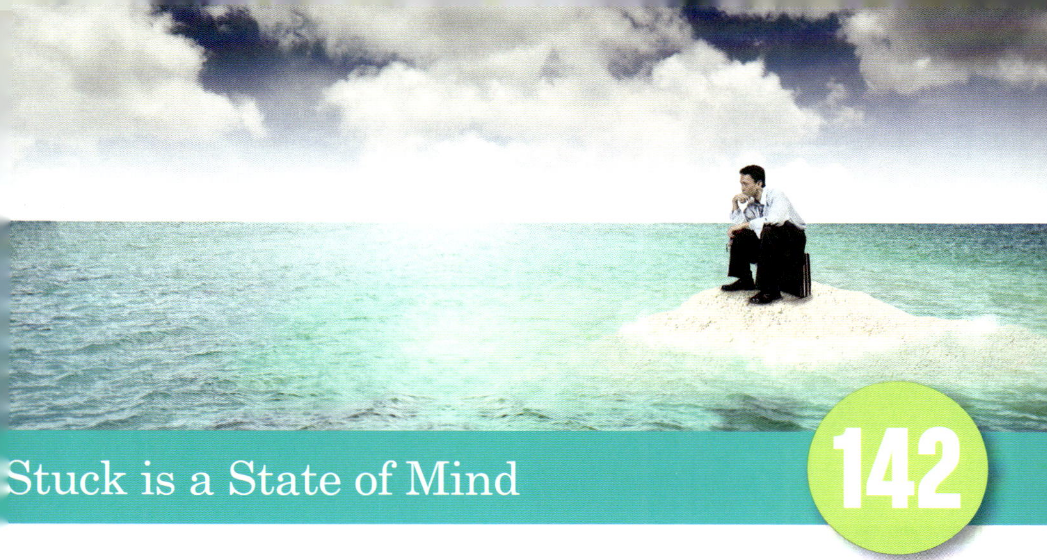

Stuck is a State of Mind

142

As I travel around the world teaching dentists how to place and restore implants, I invariably have some dentist come up to me and say some form of "I'm stuck."

- "My practice and my life are on hold."
- "I'm working harder, but enjoying it and earning less."
- "My practice has hit a plateau."
- "The insurance companies are driving me nuts, and I don't know what to do about it."
- "I never would have gotten into dentistry in the first place if I knew it was going to be like this."

Fortunately, being stuck is not caused by an overwhelming outside force. Stuck is a state of mind. All you have to do is identify what is getting in the way of you getting unstuck. There are four possibilities:

- You don't know what to do
- You don't know how to do it
- You don't have the resources to do it
- You're afraid

If you don't know what to do, do some research. Who do you know personally (or through their writings or presentations) that is unstuck to a high degree? These people tend to talk about their practices and lives in glowing terms. Listen to them and discover what they're doing.

If you don't know how to do it, learn. There are numerous educational opportunities out there where you can gain the information and skills needed to move out of your rut.

If you don't have the resources to do it, acquire them. The two most often missing resources are time and money. This is the primary reason I provide weekend implant education in many cities around the country. It lessens the time and money roadblocks to success.

If you're afraid, face your fear and do it anyway. Sure, it may be a little scary for a little while out there in the brave, new world. But that's a lot less painful than being stuck forever.

Once you figure out what's getting in your way, it's far easier to find the answer. Stuck is a state of mind, and it's curable.

CANCELLED

143 The "C-Word"

Do you ever hear comments like this in your practice?

When addressing a person at the front desk: "We don't have any time available for you next week. But don't worry. I'm sure we'll get a cancellation or two."

When confirming a visit on the phone: "If you need to cancel, please give us 24 hours notice."

I hope the words **"cancellation"** and **"cancel"** grab your attention. They are a poor choice for three reasons:

1. The words are not accurate. People usually postpone office visits. They don't cancel them.
2. The words have negative emotions attached to it.
3. They reinforce that cancellations are an accepted part of your practice.

You might be thinking right now, "This is just semantics. What difference does it really make?" You're partially right. It is just semantics… but it makes a huge difference in the messages you send. The definition of the word *semantics* is "the study of meaning in language." This is an important distinction because meaning directs thinking, creates emotion and produces action – three results not to be taken lightly.

I recommend that you enhance the two comments above:

When addressing a person at the front desk: "Can I call you at home if we have a change in our schedule where we could fit you in?"

When confirming a visit on the phone: "Hi, Bill? This is Monique from Dr. Garg's office. We're looking forward to seeing you this Friday at 11 am."

George Bernard Shaw said, "*Words are postage stamps delivering the object for you to unwrap.*" Give your patients the gift of words well chosen. They and you will benefit from the delivery.

Short.
Fast.
And to the point.

Maverick Marketing Copy (Keep it Short) 144

Whether it's an email subject line, a Facebook post, or a tweet, digital media is an increasingly truncated form of language.

Twitter only accepts 140 characters. Longer than that – in any digital format – and it's likely your audience will tune out the message.

Generally, there are several metrics to track:

For emails it's:

- **Open rate** – the number of people who open an email in a specific amount of time
- **Click-through rate** – the number of people in a given time interval who open an email and click on an offer included in the copy

For Twitter and Facebook it's:

- **Tweets and re-tweets** – the number of people who respond to your tweets by forwarding it on to someone else, furthering the online conversation
- **Shares and followers** – the number of people who share a Facebook post with a friend or colleague. The more followers you have, as with any social media (provided they're real people and not fake/automated accounts), the greater the chance more people will read and be engaged by what you post

In this world of faster, shorter, and to the point, brevity is key. Notice how this tip title is six words. A great tweet can be as short as this. Ask yourself, is what you're sending out going to inspire someone to take action? If not, chances are the metrics mentioned above will reflect that choice.

Spend time getting outreach right. Send test emails and gauge people's reactions. Remember, there are whole companies dedicated to social media metrics management. Consider reaching out to one of them, even on a limited basis, if you're serious about upping your social media game.

But even if you don't, remember shorter is better. And punchier is better still!

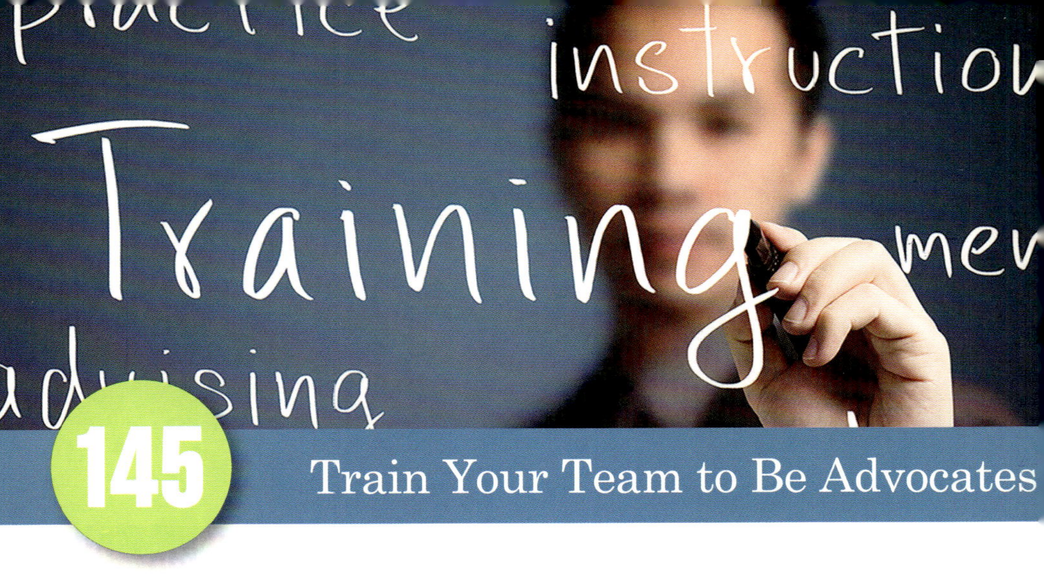

145 Train Your Team to Be Advocates

There's a saying: "The easy way is the hard way, and the hard way is the easy way." This is true when you are looking to grow your implant practice because making progress requires change – and change isn't easy! Without growth, practice profitability becomes an uphill battle.

So what types of changes are critical to growing a profitable implant practice?

One key element is changing the way you, and especially your team communicate with patients about tooth replacement options and the consequences of missing teeth.

Many times, patients trust your staff members' opinions more than yours. If there is inconsistent messaging between what you and your staff are saying, you will lose patient trust, and very likely, the case!

While an entire book can be dedicated to this topic, here we will highlight 3 tips you can apply immediately:

1. **Regular Communication:** Having regular and purposeful meetings with your team is critical. In these meetings inform and remind your staff of the direction your practice is going. Acknowledge that you have been doing things a certain way for years, and now with the evolution of dentistry, your practice is evolving too. Let them know practice growth and prosperity translates into greater opportunities for them. Also, communicate how implant dentistry changes patients' lives, and how it can be the best investment a patient can make into their health.
2. **Reward Team members:** Share success among team members. If a team member was effective in creating interest in dental implants, which led to a consultation, acknowledge their actions and offer praise. This type of recognition works wonders to keep staff motivated and promote actions that lead to practice growth.
3. **Believe in it!** If you don't believe in how you can change patients' lives with implant dentistry and the solutions you offer, how will your staff? And how will your patients? This is a domino effect that begins with you! Continue to educate yourself and communicate with colleagues and like-minded professionals about the benefits of implant dentistry. This will provide the much-needed "fuel" to energize patients and staff alike.

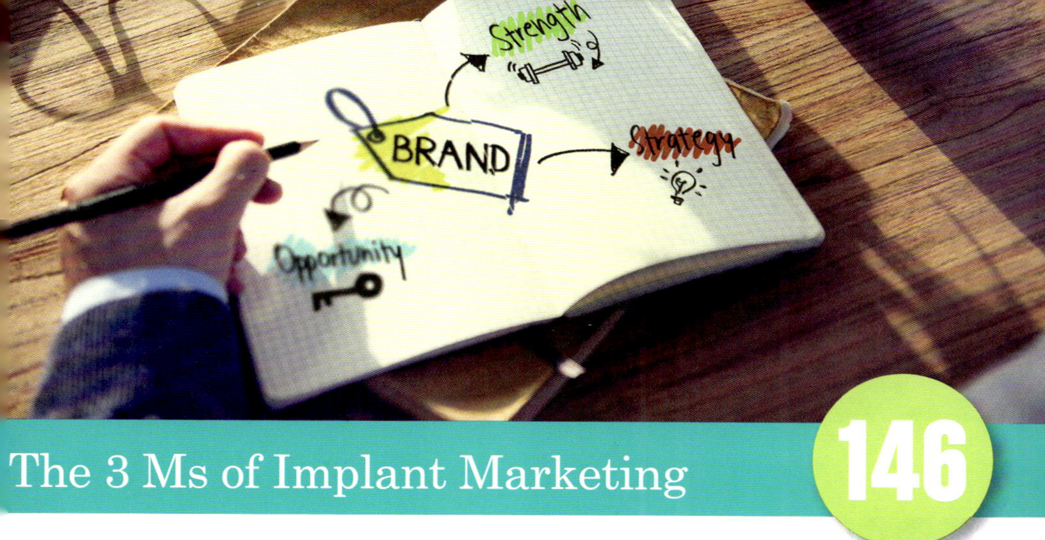

The 3 Ms of Implant Marketing

146

Follow these steps with every implant marketing program you execute to ensure your ads are more effective and profitable.

Step 1: Define your target audience – your MARKET.

Statistics show that 69% of adults ages 35 to 44 have lost at least one permanent tooth to an accident, gum disease, a failed root canal or tooth decay. By age 74, 26% of adults are fully edentulous. It's important to take such statistics into consideration – especially when defining your market. If you find most of your implant patients are between 50-70, and live in a specific part of town, then you have defined your target audience. If you find many of your patients are part of a specific retirement community – that is another target audience. The more specific your audience, the more targeted the message can become.

Step 2: Craft a MESSAGE that appeals to that target audience.

When crafting your message in your advertisements, visualize your target audience. Remember – you are literally SPEAKING to them. Understand their motivations. Use words that resonate with them. Use visuals with meaning in their lives. Mimic design styles of organizations and companies they trust and do business with.

You may also want to test drive your marketing with a few individuals in your target audience. But be sure to test drive it on someone missing teeth, or experiencing denture pain – because someone in need of your services will see your ad differently.

Step 3: Choose a MEDIA platform which can put you in front of that precise target audience

Now that you know your audience, and message, you must find the most effective media format to reach them. Align yourself with a media partner that can reach your defined audience. Avoid TV or radio unless your ads will be aligned with programs targeted to your demographic. Avoid ads in the general community paper and instead identify opportunities in targeted publications. Remember to ask all ad vendors for demographic information on readership before making any commitments.

Following the 3 steps above will help guarantee effective implant practice growth!

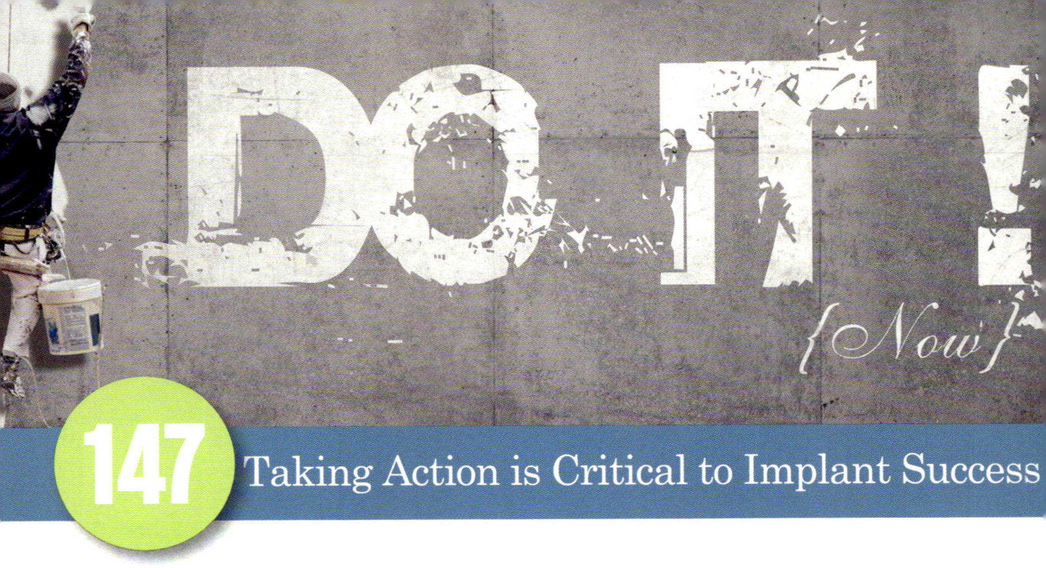

147 Taking Action is Critical to Implant Success

Offering implants to partial and fully edentulous patients can increase practice revenues by 20-30% or more. However, to do so requires more than a strategy on paper — it requires MASSIVE ACTION and execution of that strategy.

To get you started, we have included a list of ACTION items below to give you momentum as you prepare to take your practice to the next level.

1. My staff and I offer socket preservation with EVERY extraction.
   ❑ Yes ❑ No
2. My entire patient-facing staff is trained on educating patients on the benefits of implant dentistry, and how to overcome common objections patients have.
   ❑ Yes ❑ No
3. I have re-branded my practice to include "Implant Dentistry" on business cards, exterior signage, my website, and all marketing materials.
   ❑ Yes ❑ No
4. I have implemented a systematic implant case presentation tool - whether it be a PowerPoint presentation I have developed, or a patient education software I have invested in.
   ❑ Yes ❑ No
5. I have taken before and after pictures of at least 10 implant cases I've done for use in my case presentations and marketing materials.
   ❑ Yes ❑ No
6. I have acquired at least 10 patients for testimonials — either written, audio, or video — for my marketing materials.
   ❑ Yes ❑ No
7. I have met with my marketing vendor(s) to discuss and develop an implant marketing program to get the word out to patients and the community.
   ❑ Yes ❑ No
8. I have had my staff go through patient records and compile a list of edentulous patients, I can now send a target email or direct mail piece offering a complimentary consultation.
   ❑ Yes ❑ No
9. I have set a stretch goal of how many implant cases I plan to do in the next 12 months.
   ❑ Yes ❑ No

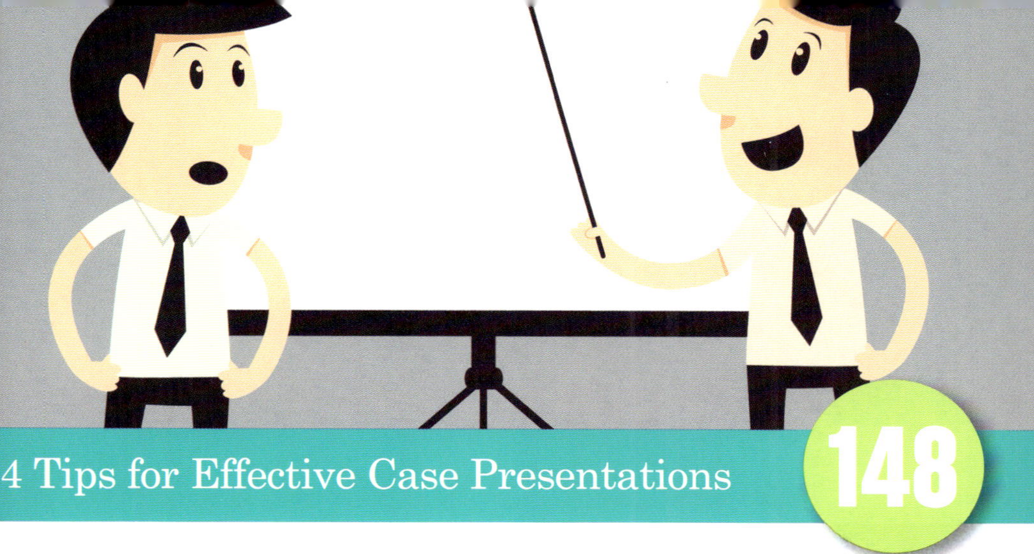

4 Tips for Effective Case Presentations

148

An effective case presentation can make all the difference between a patient saying YES or NO to your treatment plan. When you have the opportunity to deliver a case presentation, you want to do all you can to empower your patient to move forward with your treatment plan.

1. **Use a Consultation Room:** By moving discussions out of the operatory and into a consultation room you promote more effective patient-doctor communication. When patients are sitting upright in a desk chair, they feel less vulnerable and can focus better on the information at hand. You also have better control over the patient's experience in a consultation room in comparison to the many distractions which can arise in an operatory.
2. **Pay attention to Body Language during the presentation:** Effective Communication is critical when presenting implant treatment plans to patients. If you notice your patients shutting down during a case presentation or looking around the room or fidgeting then you've lost them. When this happens it's best to re-engage the patient before continuing. Try asking them a question, or ask them gently if what you are saying makes sense, or if they have any questions. Paying close attention to your patients' body language can make or break your case presentation.
3. **Provide a written treatment plan:** You may have delivered the most impressive case presentation; however, not every patient is ready to move forward immediately. It is important to recognize that many case presentations are information overload for patients and they retain 20-30% of what they have heard. For patients that are not ready to move forward with treatment it is important to provide them with a written treatment plan. Do not underestimate the power of a take-home treatment plan they can review for themselves or with a significant other. Be sure to include a brochure about dental implants that reiterates the benefit of treatment and hits on the main points discussed during your case presentation.
4. **Ask a staff member to review financial aspects of the treatment plan:** A case presentation and treatment plan proposal work best when patients feel that the doctor is focused on their oral health and not the financial aspects. For many doctors this removes them from the "conflict of interest" feeling they may have if they know at the end of the presentation they will need to discuss finances. Most well-run practices have a staff member available to manage and present the business and financial portion of treatment.

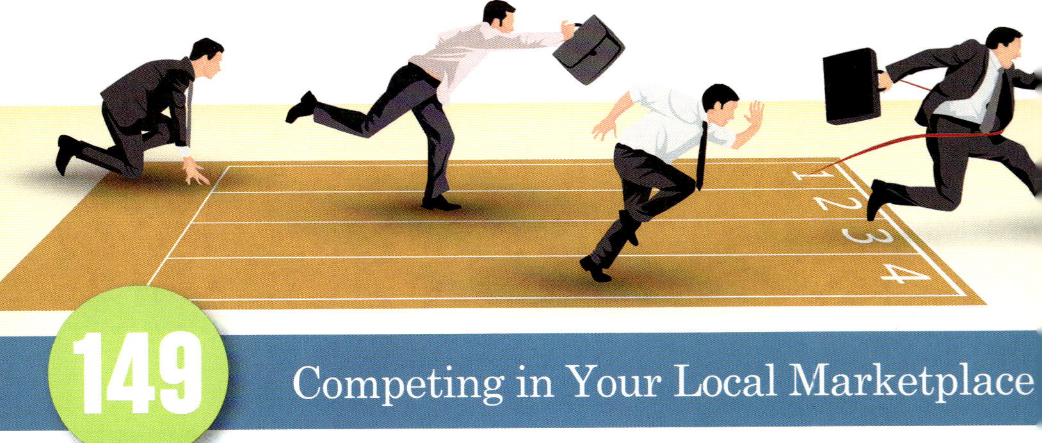

149 Competing in Your Local Marketplace

When it comes to marketing dental implants in your area, you always want to be aware of the competitive landscape — realizing patients have choice. Because of this, it is critical to conduct a review of the competition prior to developing and investing in your implant marketing campaigns.

In order to help you develop successful marketing campaigns that stand out from the crowd, we have outlined several steps below:

STEP 1: See the world through the eyes of your prospective patients. Spend 1-2 hours on Google, Yahoo, and Bing searching for "dental implants" and experience firsthand what prospective patients are seeing when they are browsing for a provider. Also, make your entire team aware of your efforts and ask them to let you know whenever they see implants advertised in newspapers and in direct mail, or on radio and television, etc. Have them bring you the ads if possible, or recount the ad details, so you get a clear picture about how other practices are positioning themselves or what they are offering to generate a response.

STEP 2: Self-test your ad. After gathering insight into your competitor's strategies and ads, ask yourself honestly: "If I was a consumer in need of implants, would I choose my practice after seeing my ad in comparison with others?" If so, great – launch your campaign, and pay attention to the campaign results to verify your conclusion. If not, you may want to reposition yourself.

STEP 3. Reposition your practice to have a competitive advantage. Make an inventory of what you can immediately offer, or what you are prepared to offer to make your ad stand out. For example if you don't compete on price — but compete on quality, security and peace of mind — then try offering some type of limited warranty or guarantee in your ad. Or consider highlighting your years of experience, amount of cases you have performed, or awards or recognitions you have. Essentially you want to highlight anything that can support your competitive advantage of providing patients with quality implants and peace of mind.

Gaining insight into your competitors will help you identify an unmet need or opportunity where you can position or reposition your practice to generate the greatest volume response for every advertising dollar spent. The greater the response, the more patients you will treat!

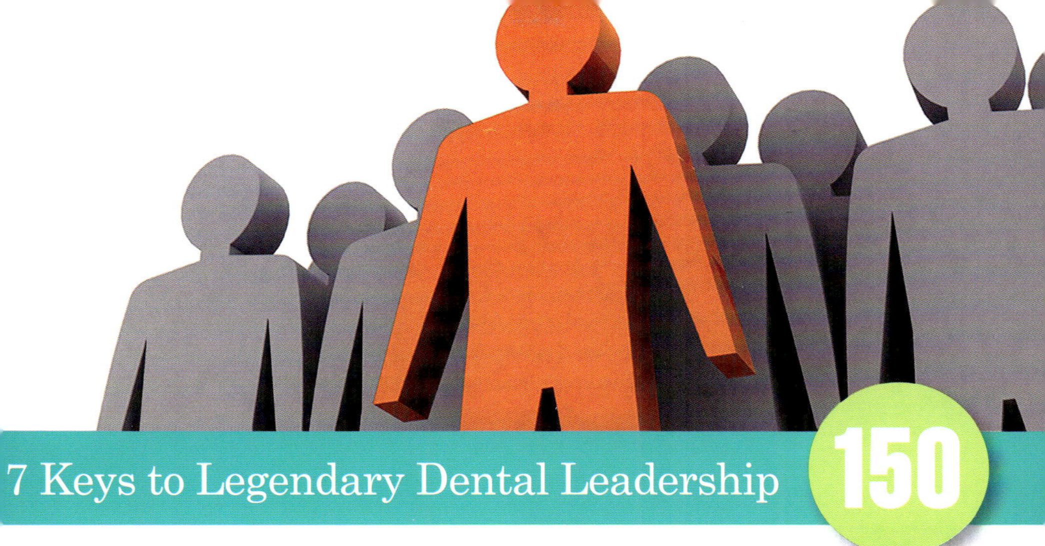

7 Keys to Legendary Dental Leadership

150

1. **Be Passionate** – Passion is created when you clearly identify a gap between where you are now and where you want to go.

2. **Build a Strong Culture** – You must hire, train and retain people who are aligned with your company's core values and the foundational principles of your practice.

3. **Understand Your Team** – The better you understand team members, the more effectively you can uniquely lead them.

4. **Bring Out the Best in Your Team** – Lead and enable your people to do their best work.

5. **Be Flexible in Leadership Styles** – Legendary leaders maximize performance by using different leadership styles for different people and situations.

6. **Improve Constantly** – Your practice is either getting better or getting worse. If you don't constantly focus on improving, it will slide in the wrong direction.

7. **Implement Effectively** – The world does not reward knowledge. It rewards action. Implementation turns your knowledge into action. Focus on these seven simple keys to help create the practice of your dreams.

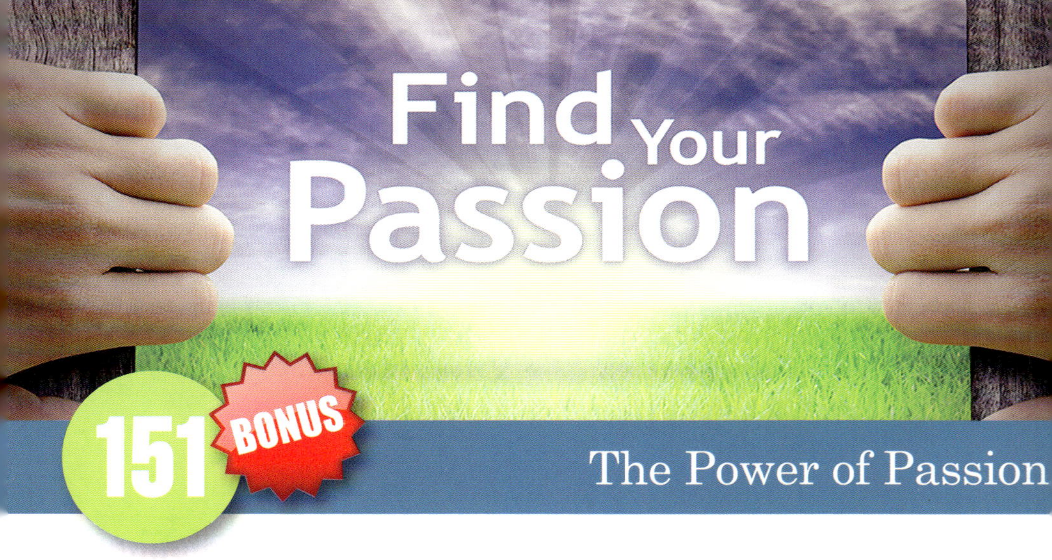

151 BONUS The Power of Passion

On a scale of 1 to 10, with 1 being a complete absence of passion, and 10 being totally passionate about building your practice, where do you fall?

Of the three types of happiness, passion is the second longest lasting. Passion occurs when peak performance meets peak engagement. When you're passionate, you're in the zone. I hope you're passionate about dentistry. Dental team members are attracted to passionate leaders. Patients are attracted to passionate dentists.

If you're not passionate about dentistry right now, examine two areas:

Peak Engagement – Peak engagement is a strong connection between your work and you. Sometimes in dentistry this engagement can weaken as the years pass. You do something enjoyable at first, but it loses its luster after a while. I'm thrilled to see the rekindling of peak engagement with my implant continuum students. They come to the first weekend of the continuum looking to recapture the excitement of our wonderful profession. By the fourth weekend, the sparkle is back in their eyes. They see how placing and restoring implants is beneficial to their patients' health and comfort… and to their mind and soul.

Peak Performance – Peak performance comes from having the training needed to do the job well, and you've done the job enough times to be unconsciously competent. So, you may need more training and/or more repetitions. I see this play out all the time with my students. The most successful ones take numerous implant courses. Then they return to their practices and take action right away. They don't think about doing it, or talk about doing it, or plan on doing it. They go back and just do it.

"Choose the job you love, and you will never have to work a day in your life."

CONFUCIUS

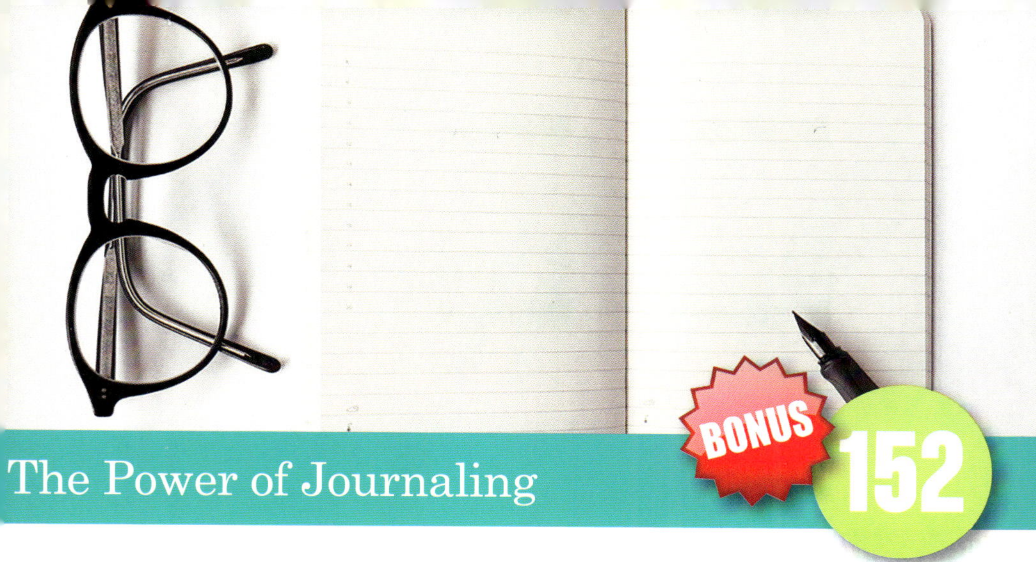

The Power of Journaling

Journaling is one of the easiest and most powerful ways to accelerate your professional and personal development. By pulling thoughts out of your head and putting them down on paper, you gain fresh and unique insights.

Your brain is capable of processing a great deal of input simultaneously, but your conscious thoughts play out in a linear sequence. Thought #1 triggers thought #2 which triggers thought #3. Like all novels and movies, these thought sequences have a beginning, a middle and an end. It's nearly impossible to see the entire sequence as you're experiencing your thoughts. Journaling allows you to break free of sequential thinking, step back and examine your thoughts in total which will bring you much closer to seeing the truth of your situation.

While many people use journaling to record a personal diary of their thoughts and experiences, the power of journaling goes way beyond verbal photography. Here are three other powerful benefits of journaling:

- **Solve problems.** Some problems are very difficult to solve when you're stuck in the first-person viewpoint. It's only when you record the situation around the problem, and then re-examine it from a third-person perspective, does the solution become clear. Sometimes the solution is so obvious that you're shocked you didn't see it sooner.
- **Gain clarity.** A great time to turn to your journal is when you're not certain about what to do. "Should I make a big change in my practice?" "What actions should my spouse and I take concerning our son who's having school challenges?" "What should I do to improve the family's financial situation?" It's amazing how much clearer things become when you explore them in writing.
- **Verify progress.** It's enlightening to go back and re-read journal entries from years past and see how much progress you've made. When you're frustrated that life doesn't seem to be working out as planned, go back and read entries written five years ago. It will totally change your perspective. Returning to the past helps you feel better in the present by reminding you of important growth you've made...even when it feels like you're stuck.

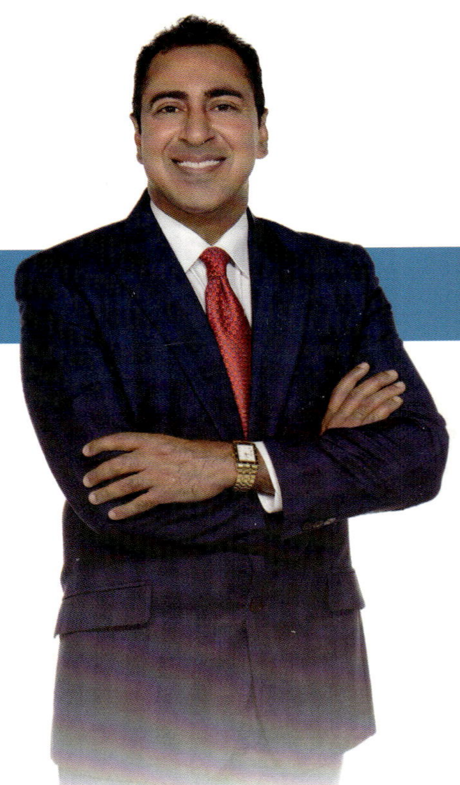

Dear Reader,

Now that you've finished reading *150 Ways to Make Your Dental Practice Rock*, I hope you appreciate the value of what I spoke about in my introduction. All it takes are minor adjustments in how you do business and how you treat your patients in order to have significant impact on your bottom line, as well as your overall dental office morale.

For your staff as much as for your patients, the dental office should be an inviting place — not an environment that causes undue anxiety or stress. I hope you found these tips timeless, informative and fun! A strong believer in transparency and a commitment to complete communication, I welcome your feedback via email and of course, on social media. If you think of additional tips, or suggestions on how to improve existing ones, don't hesitate to contact me. If you feel so inspired, send me your additions and revisions and I'll consider including them in future updates.

Dentistry truly is one of medicine's most exciting professions. Rooted in both the scientific method and the 18th and 19th century babershop trade, modern dental surgeons inherit a rich history that makes us better clinicians than academic-alone backgrounds would have provided. We are of the people and with our surgical skills, working for the people.

You may also have noticed a few extra tips beyond the 150 referenced in the title of this book. Consider the extra two tips our bonus gift to you! Why stop at 150 (other than it sounding like a nice round number, good for marketing purposes) when you can think of more? I have no doubt that in the coming years 152 tips will grow to become 160, 180 and before long 200. As technology advances and patient protocols evolve, I look forward to envisioning the dental practice of tomorrow — built on the skills and techniques learned today.

Best of luck on your continued success!

Kind regards,
Arun K. Garg, DMD